PRAISE FOR PODIATR

C000048223

Fifteen years ago, I sat in a Northeast
drinking coffee while talking on my flip phone to a guy named Rembranut.
We'd never spoken before. The purpose of the call was to see if we might
start a mutually beneficial relationship between Rem and the American
Academy of Podiatric Practice Management. We had a workshop in
Baltimore just a few days away. We arranged a meeting between our
leaders and Rem, the man who would help positively shape the direction
of our beloved Academy and its members' practices. If you're looking for
a straightforward, fun, and engaging method to bring scores of patients
to your practice, you must read this book. Every time you see Rem, he
has a new book that is a must-read—he has read every great book on
positive thinking and business and practice management ever written.
Now, he has added to that elite library with *Podiatry Prosperity: How to
Market, Manage, and Love Your Practice.*

BILL MCCANN, DPM
Concord, New Hampshire
Past president, American Academy of
Podiatric Practice Management

For any podiatrist new or old, this book is like a resident's primer—a
concise, definitive guide to marketing success. It's not only applicable in
podiatry but in any medical field or business. I thoroughly enjoyed how
it's written with an easy, step-by-step guide with quick-witted action
plans and stories that matter. I highly recommend this book.

SANJAY PATEL, DPM
Milford, Connecticut

I highly recommend *Podiatry Prosperity*. This book is your guiding light
for developing and running a successful podiatry practice at any stage.
It's a book that you'll return to again and again as you implement the
strategies and see your practice grow and become more successful. Just

as important, it will help you develop your resiliency, a much-needed life skill for practicing medicine in this challenging time.

VICTORIA L. MELHUISH, DPM
Carson City, Nevada

Podiatry Prosperity may sound like a very niche book, but once you open the pages and absorb the knowledge, you'll find that it can be transposed to any medical practice or any business. Using the information and guidance in this book, you can learn how to market and grow your practice. It's filled with important life lessons, including goal setting and how to reach your personal goals to attain success. It's a must-read for anyone who owns their own business and wants to reach the highest level of achievement.

BENJAMIN W. WEAVER, DPM
Wichita, Kansas
President, American Academy of
Podiatric Practice Management

Rem Jackson, the guru of podiatric marketing and practice building, has outdone himself this time. *Podiatry Prosperity* is the absolute must-read for all podiatric physicians on how to grow their practices into *Top Practices*. This book should catapult to the top of the podiatrist's reading list.

MICHAEL KING, DPM
Nashville, Tennessee

We receive little to no business training in our education, yet so many podiatrists are small business owners, and thus, have an unmet need. Rem Jackson has filled that need for so many of us, and his guidance applies to so much more than just a podiatry practice. Thank you, Rem, for writing this book, for what you have done for my profession, for helping so many of my colleagues, and for what you have done for me!

JEFFREY D. LEHRMAN, DPM
Springfield, Pennsylvania

"Your job is not to be a podiatrist. Your job is marketing a podiatry practice." With that simple but profound sentence, Rem Jackson changed everything I thought I knew about being a successful podiatrist. His methods, though seemingly simple and almost obvious, have helped transform my practice—and we have seen and documented exponential growth in the last seven years. Now, he has written a book outlining exactly what it takes be successful in these increasingly challenging times. For any podiatrist (and most other medical professionals) trying to survive and thrive in today's troubled times, this book should have a space on your desk and in your library.

SCOTT L. SCHULMAN, DPM
Indianapolis, Indiana

The principles and strategies found in *Podiatry Prosperity* are enduring and have withstood the test of time. They are just as relevant today as when Rem Jackson first introduced them in 2007. I know from personal experience that if you follow Rem's Four Pillars of Marketing, your practice will be guaranteed success and will thrive.

JENNY L. SANDERS, DPM
San Francisco, California

Podiatry Prosperity will ultimately guide and influence you in ways you can only imagine. My journey with Rem and Top Practices started in 2009, when I hired my first associate. Now ten years later, we have four physicians and a nurse practitioner working in a 6,800-square-foot office. This kind of growth was made possible through the marketing lessons and coaching provided in this book. This book is a special gift to our profession.

JANE E. GRAEBNER, DPM
Delaware, Ohio

Owning, operating, or working for a podiatry practice can be hard, lonely, and even unrewarding. Loving it is harder yet. Thriving in such a practice personally, financially, and spiritually seems, to many, almost impossible. But to Rem Jackson, these are the things of his every day work and life. In *Podiatry Prosperity*, he discloses a lifetime of learning, from teaching to helping podiatrists to achieve success in all aspects of their practices and their lives. This book is real, proven, and practical strategy and advice. It's not just *what* to do; it's *how* to do it. Get this book and thrive.

DAVE FREES
Attorney and author
Phoenixville, Pennsylvania

Podiatry Prosperity lays out the principles to follow when marketing your podiatry practice. These fundamentals have been tested and refined over many years to bring you the latest and best techniques to use. Rem Jackson has defined the way marketing should be. Following these principles and ideas can be an asset to any practice.

HARVEY DANCIGER, DPM
Palm Desert, California

The title of this book suggests that prosperity in podiatry is the goal. That's true, but it's much more than that. It's about taking a hard look into the scary part of owning a very successful practice. That means learning business, something most of us don't know much about. Or we think we can run a business, but we don't have much guidance. While working through the Four Pillars of Marketing, Rem Jackson gives pertinent suggestions and recommendations that can be used right away. This is a fun and easy book to read and will make you want more.

DOCK DOCKERY, DPM
Director, International Foot & Ankle Foundation
Seattle, Washington

Rem Jackson has been on a mission to improve the lives of podiatrists for over a decade. *Podiatry Prosperity* encourages you to think and visualize the type of practice you really want—one that works for you, rather than you working for it. It's not just a book about building your practice; it's a book about building your life.

TONY ABBOTT, CHIROPODIST
Collingwood, Ontario, Canada

Rem Jackson teaches effective and consistent marketing tools that will take your practice to whatever level you desire. He teaches time-tested business concepts that anyone can apply. There are always obstacles in private practice, but Rem will show you how those obstacles can be overcome by a change in mindset. *Podiatry Prosperity* is a must-read for those podiatrists who wonder how to thrive in private practice instead of just treading water.

KEVIN F. SUNSHEIN, DPM
Dayton, Ohio

I'm proud and grateful to know Rem Jackson. Time and time again, I've witnessed Rem leading doctors to increased wealth and happiness. Initially, success is clearly defined. Once defined, Rem provides direction to stop doing certain things and start doing what it takes to be successful.

ROBERT BLAINE, DPM
CEO and Founder Blaine Labs

I've been a coaching client of Rem Jackson's, as well as a member of Top Practices, for over ten years. *Podiatry Prosperity* is a must-read for every podiatry student and practicing podiatrist in the country. Rem's sage advice has changed the course of my life and will change yours, too, if you choose to listen.

MARYBETH CRANE, DPM
Grapevine, Texas

Hooray for Rem Jackson! He's hit it out of the ballpark with this book. In trying to learn marketing for my practice of twenty-nine years, I always had to resort to books written by dentists, chiropractors, and medical doctors. There's never been an extensive book about marketing and productivity for podiatrists. This book is long overdue for our profession. Don't put this book on your shelf, expecting to read it later. Open it up right now, and when you're finished, go back and re-read it while taking notes. Leave this book on your desk to refer to anytime you need help. The information within is priceless, and it will help you make more money while being more productive.

PETER A. WISHNIE, DPM
Director of Physician Programming
Top Practices Virtual Practice Management Institute
Piscataway, New Jersey

Fantastic work from a fantastic man who has personally helped me wade through some very difficult waters in my practice. If you internalize, act on, and execute only a fraction of what Rem offers in this book, it will revolutionize your practice!

ERIC WILLIAMS, MD
Baltimore, Maryland

Rem Jackson lives, eats, and breathes podiatry marketing, and *Podiatry Prosperity* is a testament to all the years of hard work that he's put into helping podiatrists own and operate more successful and profitable podiatry businesses. If you only apply part of what you read in this book, your business will be better for it. But if you apply the whole book, it will change your thinking, life, and podiatry business forever.

TYSON FRANKLIN, PODIATRIST
Cairns, Queensland, Australia

This book contains all the ingredients needed to successfully market a practice. Once you add the "5th" pillar, which is Rem Jackson, you'll be guaranteed success. The information spelled out in *Podiatry Prosperity* has taken my practice from good to great and still growing. Thank you, Rem, for all your help and knowledge.

KEVIN S. MOLAN, DPM
Charlotte, North Carolina

Rem Jackson could have easily named this book The Secrets of Success instead of *Podiatry Prosperity*. If you wonder why some practices succeed and others fail, this is the book for you. Rem outlines in a straightforward, easy-to-read format the principles that each practice needs to take. I've seen Rem turn average doctors into highly successful practitioners. If you want to be successful and would like to begin the journey making your practice what you have always dreamed of, this book is the place to start.

JEFFREY FREDERICK, DPM
Past President, American Academy of
Podiatric Practice Management and
Executive Vice President, NEMO Health

Rem Jackson has been guiding recently graduated and established podiatrists into the new age of marketing for many years now. His lectures, written word, and hallway hoedowns have enlightened all and led to many ultra-successful podiatric practices. Rem loves life and all its amenities, and it shows in his ability to guide those of us in need of podiatric practice management skills.

CHARLES GREINER, DPM
Portsmouth, Ohio

Rem Jackson is a marketing guru. He has personally transformed my practice over the past six years with these *exact* techniques and methods. This allowed me to build the practice I want, not the one I have to accept. This book will become an annual must-read for me as it should for any podiatric entrepreneur who wants to grow and enrich their practice and their lives. Well done, Rem!

MELISSA LOCKWOOD, DPM
Bloomington, Illinois

Rem Jackson is the real thing. What you see and hear is what you really get. He's one of the most genuine, caring people that I've had the opportunity to work with and to know as a friend. Time and time again, when I speak with the physicians and staff who've worked with Rem and Top Practices, they sing nothing but praises and have sincere gratitude for how he puts them first and wants the best for them and their practice. We are blessed that Rem landed in the podiatry field and has invested in growing our profession with ethical standards and high integrity.

TINA DEL BUONO, PMAC
Director, Top Practices Virtual
Practice Management Institute
Santa Rose, California

Rem Jackson is a fixture at podiatry conferences across the country. A master communicator, he's able to break down the nuances of marketing a medical practice and present them in such a way that every attendee walks away with an action plan. In *Podiatry Prosperity*, Rem packages the enthusiasm he has on the stage and brings it to the page. Readers will be entertained by this easy-to-read book but will also find themselves going back to refer to the many pearls of wisdom ready to be immediately implemented in their practice. I highly recommend *Podiatry Prosperity* to any practitioner looking to explode their practice and embrace their success.

ANDREW SCHNEIDER, DPM
Houston, Texas

Rem Jackson quite possibly saved my marriage. My wife and I thought we were running our practice, but in reality, it was running us. We were helplessly adrift in the currents of business without a paddle, a rudder, or any navigation. Rem and Top Practices gave us direction, advice, and a compass, and then they taught us the principles necessary to take control of our business. Rem also empowered us with this quote from Napoleon Hill: "Whatever the mind can conceive and believe, it can achieve." I'm happy to say that we've since traded that leaky canoe for a frigate! This book distills all the strategies and processes we used to significantly increase our practice, down to a usable blueprint for practice growth and prosperity. Highly recommended!

GREGG NEIBAUER, DPM
Missoula, Montana

The ideas and personal inspiration gathered from Rem Jackson have been immensely helpful, not only to me, but to my patients and support staff as well. Mr. Jackson has and will continue to have a positive influence with the release of his book for the podiatric and other professions for many years to come.

LAWRENCE KALES, DPM
Bayonet Point, Florida

In *Podiatry Prosperity*, you'll learn how to grow your practice by using clearly defined marketing pillars. This deceptively simple formula has allowed my financial and operational performance to improve year over year! Rem Jackson and his program have transformed my practice by providing a roadmap and the key actions needed to build my practice through great marketing. Everything I do to continue to grow my practice is supported by the solutions in this book.

CRAIG H. THOMAJAN, DPM
Austin, Texas

PODIATRY
PROSPERITY

REM JACKSON

PODIATRY
PROSPERITY

HOW TO
MARKET, MANAGE,
AND
LOVE YOUR PRACTICE

REM JACKSON

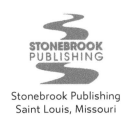

Stonebrook Publishing
Saint Louis, Missouri

To Diane

Emily, Annie, Iris

CONTENTS

FOREWORD

In 2007, I met a man who would eventually change my mindset and that of my podiatry colleagues and who set many of us on a pathway to success, despite the tumultuous decade that was ahead. Since that time, what it takes to practice medicine successfully has changed considerably, yet this man always seemed to have the answers. He never viewed an obstacle as a problem but, rather, saw it as a challenge that could easily be overcome if you combined the right mindset along with proven strategies.

As the years passed, I grew to truly love and respect this man. He has an unwavering passion for helping others and lives his life just as he preaches. It's apparent that I'm not the only one who holds this sentiment. He was recently inducted into *Podiatry Management's* prestigious Podiatric Hall of Fame by our profession. I'm excited that you are about to read his book and join the many that he's made successful!

Rem Jackson could potentially change your life. You might change the way you view yourself, the way you approach challenges, the way you view success, and the way you grow professionally. In fact, each reader will probably benefit in a different way, but one thing is for sure: you *will* grow personally and professionally by reading Rem's story, learning from his poignant anecdotes, and following his recipe for success.

In this book and throughout his lectures and presentations, Rem refers to "pillars" of success. He's created a unique and easy-to-follow formula to grow your podiatry practice, no matter what challenges are thrown your way. As you read this book, keep in mind what a pillar represents—a monument of strength and support. That image clearly represents what Rem Jackson has accomplished for the podiatry profession throughout his years of teaching and now in this new and exciting book. I urge you to not only read it, but study it, re-read it, live it, and breathe it, just as Rem does. Your life will change!

Happy and successful reading, my fellow colleagues!

JOHN V. GUILIANA, DPM, MS
Executive Vice President, NEMO Health

TOP PRACTICES

In times of change, the learners will inherit the earth; while the learned find themselves beautifully equipped to deal with a world that no longer exists.

—ERIC HOFFER

Let's face it; you're a podiatrist. You've invested and sacrificed more to practice podiatry than most people will ever invest in their careers, and you're one of the most educated people on the planet. And yet, when you went to podiatry school, you probably didn't think too much about all the non-medical aspects of practicing this profession. Who would spend all those years in education and training to ultimately deal with ridiculous federal regulations, overbearing intrusion by payers, and all the unique complications that small businesses face? No, these frustrations seemed to appear out of nowhere while you were minding your own business and practicing medicine. Had you known how crippling they could be, you might have considered doing something else.

But you're a podiatrist—and that's a wonderful thing.

The good news is that you can be happy and extremely successful in this profession. You *can* and *will* experience prosperity and abundance as a podiatrist if you know how and if you want it enough.

- If you know how to market and manage your practice

- If you want to earn the income you know you deserve and can maintain a mindset that will change your life

- If you want your nights and weekends back

In fact, you can accomplish everything you want in life through the incredible vehicle of your podiatry practice.

This is serious business.

But before I tell you how you can do that, you should know my story to gain some insight into how Top Practices came to be.

I had a slow start after I graduated from Penn State University with a political science degree. I had planned to go to law school and was accepted to five good schools, but I had a problem. I'd interned with a lawyer for one semester and realized that I didn't like anything about the actual *practice* of law. When I read case law, I almost immediately got distracted because I couldn't get interested in the material. Contracts have always been hard for me to read, and they still are. I later learned that contracts could be very interesting and even fun for some people like my daughter, Iris, who's an attorney. She loves everything about her work.

But not me.

Without any plans or goals or even a sense of what I wanted, I drifted for a few years. After some soul-searching and growth, I took a job at a small publishing company, and a colleague, Diane Whitman, was charged with teaching me how to use the computer. Whip-smart, shy, and reserved, and with a great sense of humor, she taught me the DOS computer system, and I fell in love with her. After many lunches and coffee breaks, always with an eye not to screw it up with her, we had our first date and have now been married for almost thirty years.

Even a blind squirrel gets a nut every once in a while!

Together we created an unstoppable team. Her smarts and my communication skills worked well together, and I quickly rose in the ranks of the company where we worked. She had all the good ideas, and I sold them. When our company's high-tech education initiative, Classroom Connect, sold to venture capitalists, they asked us to move to Southern California to run the professional development programs. Diane and I jumped at the chance, and we packed up our three young daughters and moved to Los Angeles.

Now sure that I would learn how "the big dogs" ran companies, I discovered that they had the same problems we had at a little company. The only real difference was the size of the numbers. More money, more people, same problems. I would sit in the room with brilliant people and as they worked on our business issues. I often thought that the plans they made seemed destined to fail for one reason or another, but I didn't say anything because they surely knew more than me. It all seemed to make sense to them. But as time went by, all the things I'd worried about came to pass.

My division continued to prosper and grow. Always responsible with our venture investments, my group continued to grow our part of the business. The larger company, however, continued to burn through a remarkable amount of cash. That, in conjunction with the stalled market in K-12 technology education, caught up with us, and the company began to fail. I left with a golden parachute and ample time to contemplate my next move.

After one last attempt to work with a small K-12 company that turned Game Boys and Palm Pilots into instructional devices—impractical but cool—Diane and I returned to Lancaster, Pennsylvania to work with professionals (doctors and lawyers) as we had so many years ago when we first met. But you can't go home. That effort failed after eighteen months because of a big difference in vision between the guys I worked with and me.

I finally got some clarity. I'd come to trust in my judgment and realized I'd only be truly happy when I was the CEO of my own company. But that meant I'd have to start my own company, which I found extremely intimidating.

By nature, I'm pretty conservative and to jump out into this entrepreneurial world without a safety net scared me. But I had no choice. I simply had to do it, and several things made it possible. First, I'd met with a group of podiatrists six months earlier, The Board of Trustees of the American Academy of Podiatric Practice Management (AAPPM), who were focused on sharing the very best ideas they could find to help their fellow podiatrists succeed. From them, I learned that podiatrists needed marketing and management ideas, and they needed help implementing those ideas. Second, I'd learned a much better way of marketing than I'd ever even seen before, and I knew it worked. I knew I had a solid solution. Third, I shared the whole idea with Diane, who's always told me exactly what she thinks.

She looked me right in the eyes and said, "I think you have a great idea."

She believed in me both professionally and personally, and she was all in. She also thought I needed her full-time support and partnership to pull it off, and she was ready to work in this new venture with me. If Diane hadn't offered those encouraging words and meant them, I don't think I would've had the courage to pull the trigger. Our twin daughters were soon to be on their way to college, plus we already had one daughter pursuing her degree.

Finally, my best friend since childhood listened to my idea. I respected his opinion for many reasons, one being that he was in the process of selling his own company quite successfully. Although he didn't quite understand my business model, he had the same firm belief in me as Diane had, and he stood behind me all the way.

So, I did it. And it worked.

I was prepared to run my own company the right way with a true vision of what great marketing is with my fantastic partner who completed me as I did her. Diane and I launched Top Practices on January 2, 2007. We had the idea for a company, and we had a method that would help doctors grow their practices. We also had some strategic relationships and a mastermind alliance of good, like-minded people who were growing their companies as we grew ours. So, we took flight.

When I finally made that leap, I realized that the safety net I thought I'd had when I worked for others *actually put me in a cage*. Now that I owned my own business with my smart, beautiful wife beside me, I found the freedom I desired.

I've always believed that if something is supposed to work, it just works. Top Practices worked. The company has grown every year and continues to thrive. I believe our growth is directly related to how much we're able to help our members. The more we help, the more we grow. As long as we all strive to serve our customers, clients, or patients better and more deeply, we will grow. The moment we forget that, we stop growing.

I will never again think of a J.O.B. as something I should have. I'm more than willing to trade the hard life of an entrepreneur and business owner for the rewards of risks, failures, and more risks. I want every doctor who reads this book to know they have bestowed an invaluable gift upon themselves: their business. No one can take that freedom, that power to earn, and that satisfaction from you. Only you have the power to do that. This book is written for the sole purpose to teach you the tools and strategies you need to be your own best supporter and to have your small business flourish.

> THIS BOOK IS WRITTEN FOR THE SOLE PURPOSE TO TEACH YOU THE TOOLS AND STRATEGIES YOU NEED TO BE YOUR OWN BEST SUPPORTER AND TO HAVE YOUR SMALL BUSINESS FLOURISH.

Of course, that doesn't mean there won't be heartbreak along the way. The hardest ship to sail is a *partnership*. That's why I've only had one business partner, Diane, which has been a joy and a privilege every day. I have, however, had many strategic alliances. Some of them are treasures and endure to this day. Others, some of my closest and most important, have been heartbreaking lessons in misunderstandings, betrayals, and loss of close relationships. Even so, I'm grateful for all those relationships, regardless of how they ended.

I'm lucky that Top Practices can operate from anywhere that has a good airport and an internet connection. A couple of years ago, Diane and I moved twelve miles west and one thousand feet higher than the Las Vegas strip to the Mojave Desert, just outside of Red Rock Canyon.

I call that happily ever after.

Every morning when I open the window shades and the relentless desert sunlight streams in my windows, I'm grateful for the gifts of entrepreneurship. I'm grateful for my partner. I'm grateful for my doctors and their staffs, who are our clients. I have my morning coffee, head to my office, and try to serve my doctor members to my utmost. It's a nice way to spend a good day.

This book is the culmination of what I've learned over a decade of "in the trenches" tried-and-true strategies and tactics that can help you to weather any storm that comes your way while enjoying the ride.

Let's get started.

PROSPERITY TIPS:

- Trust your inner voice. It's smarter than you think and will serve you well.

- Your close, personal relationships, including that with your spouse, are your most important assets. Take care of these relationships.

- You are a podiatrist. Thank yourself every day for the sacrifices you've made for this privilege to serve. Resolve to make your practice the best-run practice in the country.

DISCUSSION QUESTIONS:

- How do you access your own inner voice? How often do you ignore it? How often is it right?

- What do you do to protect, nurture, and grow your relationship with your spouse/significant other?

- How can you reinforce an attitude of gratefulness for your chosen career on a daily basis?

THE FOUR PILLARS OF MARKETING

Personally, I am very fond of strawberries and cream, but I have found that for some strange reason, fish prefer worms.

—DALE CARNEGIE

t's pretty simple. There are only four places that direct patients to you, and they are:

- The internet

- Medical and non-medical referral sources

- Your own list (database) of people who know you, like you, and trust you

- The community, through advertising and other marketing efforts

That's it. There's nowhere else that patients come from. We call the marketing plan that we use ourselves at Top Practices and use to guide our clients The Four Pillars of Marketing.

THE FOUR PILLARS OF MARKETING

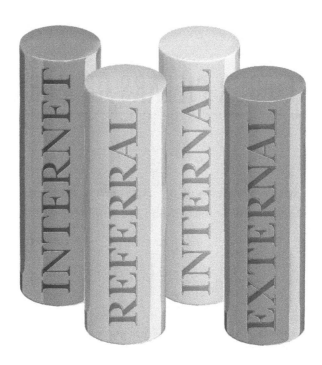

Here's the thing—no pillar is more important than any of the others. You must use all four. And yet, people sometimes fall in love with one pillar and focus all their marketing efforts on that. In fact, many marketing companies that serve medical practices seem to believe that internet marketing is the only game in town. Not so.

Internet marketing *is* important to your marketing mix and is very effective, but it's not all there is to professional practice marketing. When you understand this one vital concept, you'll outperform anyone, anywhere, anytime, no matter how big their budget is.

MARKETING YOUR BUSINESS SHOULD BE FUN. IT SHOULD *ALWAYS* BE PROFITABLE.

Marketing your business should be fun. It should *always* be profitable. If you understand what good marketing looks like, and if you have the mindset you need to persist, you'll have more fun, make more money, and find more freedom than you

8

ever dreamed your practice could bring you, your family, your staff, and your patients.

Pillar #1: Internet Marketing

In 1994, I worked for an educational technology company named Classroom Connect. At that time, most people hadn't yet heard about the internet. It remained the domain of university folks, the military, librarians, and people who would later be very proud to be called geeks.

IBM was running a commercial that showed two businessmen at breakfast with newspapers in their hands as they sipped their morning coffee. One looked up and said to the other one, "It says here we should have our business on the internet."

The other man looked up and said, "Why?"

The first guy looked back at his paper for a moment, looked back up, and said, "It doesn't say." They both shrugged and went back to their papers.

A lot has happened since then, but for many medical practices (and most professionals and a lot of businesses) their online presence and reputation isn't much further along than those guys back in 1994.

These days, almost everyone has a website. In fact, that seems to be one of the first things in everyone's business plans: a good website with search engine optimization (SEO), whatever that means to them. And many of these websites are beautiful and delight their owners, but if they aren't viewed by anyone, then they are a useless vanity expense.

There's only one reason to have a website, a Facebook page, a Pinterest page, or any other online tool, and that's effective communication with people who have problems, worries, or needs that you can solve.

You have a website to make money.

If your website can't be found by people who are searching for answers to the questions that keep them up at night, then it's worthless.

Luckily for all of us, Google appointed themselves the "sheriff" of the internet and has worked tirelessly and brilliantly to maintain the integrity of online search—not a guaranteed outcome when Tim Berners-Lee invented the World Wide Web in 1989.

IF YOUR WEBSITE CAN'T BE FOUND BY PEOPLE WHO ARE SEARCHING FOR ANSWERS TO THE QUESTIONS THAT KEEP THEM UP AT NIGHT, THEN IT'S WORTHLESS.

Tim Berners-Lee is one of my personal heroes. He's a British engineer and computer scientist who worked in Switzerland at the CERN facility. And as often happens, to make his job easier, he invented a tool: hypertext. It was a way that documents could point to other documents on a network. And that became the World Wide Web when he *gave it away* to humanity to do what we would with it. He didn't trademark or patent hypertext—he just gave it to humanity with no strings or costs attached. Every website you've ever seen, including your own, is a gift from this scientist. He changed the world.

Then Google showed up after many other search engines fell by the wayside, and they've been relentless in protecting the quality of search. And we spend a significant amount of time trying to guess Google's algorithms that produce search results. We call this *search engine optimization* (SEO). It's not that hard to understand Google because they tell us what constitutes good search techniques. It astounds me how rarely this is well understood by companies who claim that they know good SEO for doctors. They should be able to do this well. The truth is that it takes discipline and vigilance and adaptability to be good at SEO, and that always seems to be in low supply.

Google went on to develop sophisticated user analytics that track everything that happens on every page of every website that has Google Analytics enabled, and these analytics are a treasure trove of information you can use. Google did this for their own purposes but had the foresight to make some of it available to all of us so that, using this information, we could improve the performance of our websites.

Make sure that Google Analytics is enabled on every page of your website.

Look at the reports Google provides, and learn how to read them. Do it monthly. If your digital marketing company can't or won't provide you with this information, and if they won't work with you to understand your website analytics, then hire another company. And if they have their own proprietary analytics they prefer to use, politely thank them and then demand Google Analytics. In Google Analytics we trust!

There's a danger when I write about the most important features, reports, and numbers you should review and the strategies you should pursue when armed with this information because it changes almost every day. Google and all the other search engines are in constant war with the rest of humanity who try to trick their algorithms, so they continually refine and change those algorithms to maintain the integrity of their search. I will share the essentials with you. My goal is to give you the information you need to make informed decisions about who will do this work for you.

MAKE SURE THAT GOOGLE ANALYTICS IS ENABLED ON EVERY PAGE OF YOUR WEBSITE.

First, let's talk about pretty websites. I'm not against them. In fact, your website needs to be designed to be congruent with your branding—colors, logos, everything—but it needs to be much more than merely pretty.

Websites are like cars in many ways. The reason we have cars is to take us places we want to go when we want to go there. And even though cars have one function, to move us, we spend an excessive amount of time and effort selecting them.

We obsess over the body, the maker, the color, and all those extra features. We identify with our cars. We project status onto our precious vehicles, and we frequently trade them in.

Diane and I bought a sharp little Lexus convertible, a gorgeous blue color, which looked like some kind of car of the future whenever we put the top up or down. It gleamed like a work of art. But it's a good thing we aren't into performance because it didn't have a very peppy engine. Not terrible, but let's just say it wasn't a thrill to accelerate on a freeway on-ramp.

You can buy a beautiful car, but if it's powered by an engine better suited for a lawnmower, it won't do you much good. It's the same with websites. If your website is beautiful but no one can find it, it's useless. And here's the problem—without your analytics and reports, you don't know how effective it is. The ultimate report card for your online marketing, of which your website is the centerpiece, is how many patients are in your reception room each and every day.

Doctors don't know how to evaluate their online marketing, and this has made them targets for the new "snake-oil" salesman: digital marketing companies. Hundreds have sprung up over the past five years, and they are all "experts" in marketing medical practices. The problem is that they aren't expert at much except for separating doctors from their money. It can be very difficult to sort out the truth with these companies.

Consider these questions as you evaluate who can get you the right results for the right money:

- Who do your smart colleagues work with?

- What firms specialize in podiatry?

- How long have they been in business, specifically in podiatry?

- Can they give you multiple great references? And are those references featured on their own website?

- Can they show you dozens and dozens of great testimonials?

- When you search for podiatry marketing companies, do they show up?

To evaluate your current company:

- Conduct the kinds of searches your patients would use in your market. Use the *incognito search function* of your browser so it doesn't recognize you and skew your results.

- If your marketing company writes content for you and publishes it online, copy several paragraphs and paste it into your browser to see if it appears on other websites. If it does, then your company has disqualified themselves and must be replaced. Duplicate content on multiple websites is one of the best ways to have Google drop you lower and lower in their search results. If your current company knows this, then shame on them. If they don't know it, shame on them again.

- Does the marketing company answer the phone when you call, or do they call you right back?
- Do they meet with you to review your results online, and do they work with you to get content they can use to promote you?

Your website is your home online. It's the heart of all your marketing. Everything you do online should direct your prospects to call your office to get more information or make an appointment.

A well-designed website is easy to use and understand. It has offers that are easy to find for extended information, like books that viewers can either download or request that go into more detail about how you serve your patients. A great website has testimonials from happy patients you've helped and great videos that answer questions and introduce you to the viewers, so that when they come to see you, they feel like they already know you.

Well-designed websites have one goal—converting prospects to patients. They accomplish this through education, reassurance, and building a connection. The online offers are designed to extend the relationship and to capture the viewer's contact information so they can be integrated into your marketing database and then marketed to in a variety of ways.

> WELL-DESIGNED WEBSITES HAVE ONE GOAL—CONVERTING PROSPECTS TO PATIENTS. THEY ACCOMPLISH THIS THROUGH EDUCATION, REASSURANCE, AND BUILDING A CONNECTION.

Remember, the reason to have a website is to find new patients and serve your current patients better.

A website that's inexpensive and does nothing is an especially bad choice for two reasons. First, it lulls you into complacency because you've checked the "I've got a website" box and nothing happens. Second, it produces nothing when it's a marketing pillar that can be one of the best and most lucrative investments you can make in your practice. Don't scrimp on your website.

Here's my personal philosophy: in life, there are three things you should never ever scrimp on. The first is your pillow. I spent $500 on the two pillows I sleep on every night. $500 per pillow! Yep, my head rests on $1,000 worth of pillows every night. And I would pay twice that for those pillows.

Sometime in mid-life, I became sensitive and obsessed with my pillows. I couldn't care less about the bed as long as the pillows are good. That's just me, but when I found these pillows, I started sleeping well. I spend eight hours a night sleeping, which is so important. Why would I scrimp? Diane looked shocked when she found out how much I paid for these pillows, but since I was leaving for a business trip right after they came, I suggested she try them out. The next morning, I got a text from her that said, "Buy me a pillow."

Second, never scrimp on your computer monitor. Get the biggest, baddest, most awesome monitor you can find. Or get three. To squint for half your life is not an option. Why would any sane person save their money in this area if they work every day on their computer screen as I do? I don't know, do you?

Finally, never scrimp on your marketing. Marketing, websites, and everything you do to promote your practice, if done well, is an investment that will return more to you than any other investment you can make.

Why would you get a cheap website that no one can find, and if they do find it, it doesn't represent you well? Your marketing, like your pillow, is an investment in your health and happiness. When it comes to digital marketing, make your website a budget priority. Work with people who support you, and over time, you'll see your reception room filled with precisely the kind of patients you'd like to treat every day.

Every single home run hitter we've coached in Top Practices has spent the money to make a great website, and not one of them regrets it.

I consider it my mission to protect Top Practices' members from the misunderstandings and misleading services sold online. We are happy to recommend specific companies and, of course, we also do this work ourselves for our members.

But internet marketing can't help you if you don't have five-star reviews on all possible review sites. These days, reviews matter as much as anything. Let's look at why.

LOCAL LISTINGS AND REVIEWS

Sometimes, you have to take a stand against something. Since 2007, I've taken a stand against the Yellow Pages. I've been predicting their demise for years. In 2007, the Yellow Pages had a strongly entrenched position, and no one would consider pulling their ads from them. The writing was on the wall even then, but it took a few more years of my evangelizing to take down the Yellow Pages all by myself. Which I did. (Well, I did have a little help from Google.)

Please don't get me wrong; the Yellow Pages had their day. Once upon a time, the very best way to tell people about your business was through this big book filled with phone numbers and advertisements. All the way through the last century, the Yellow Pages was the only significant game in town. But when was the last time you browsed through that book?

A few years ago, one of our doctors met a Yellow Pages rep to tell him that he wasn't going to spend all that money with them anymore. The YP rep asked the doctor if he liked his bike, which he almost always rode to work.

He answered, "Yes. Why?"

"That's good," the rep said, "because you won't be able to afford your BMW after you do this."

I think they used to send YP reps to Doctor Intimidation School to teach those kinds of tactics. These days, they tell you that they'll do all the internet marketing for you—and they do—but why would you trust your internet marketing to a giant company who treats you the same way they treat party rental companies, plumbers, and dry cleaners? It doesn't make sense. I used to wonder how it would all shake out, and then Google got very interested in local search, which has become a crucial part of their business model.

Google killed the Yellow Pages. Of course, YP online made some last-gasp efforts, but again, Google made them irrelevant. Dinosaurs had their day and went extinct, and now it's YP's turn.

Your local footprint online—directories, Yelp, Healthgrades®, Rate MDs, Google, and many other directories that list your practice—is as important as your excellent website. Perhaps even more important because people will often interact with those things first. And yet, if your local search sends them to a disappointing and ineffective website, then it doesn't matter how good your local search is. People will still go somewhere else. But you've already taken the time to invest in a great website, so let's talk about why your local search is so critical.

That's simple: It's how people find you today. Local search is where they check you out most frequently, and it's often where they make a key decision based on your online reputation.

LOCAL SEARCH IS WHERE THEY CHECK YOU OUT MOST FREQUENTLY. AND IT'S OFTEN WHERE THEY MAKE A KEY DECISION BASED ON YOUR ONLINE REPUTATION.

There are a remarkable number of directories, search engines, and social media platforms that include you and your practice, whether you know it or not, or whether you even care. They share the basic information such as where your office is located, your hours of operation, your contact information (which could be incorrect), your photo, and reviews that people have posted online. This information must be up to date, accurate, and engaging. It's impossible to try to find all these listings through searches or by trying to do this manually.

Marketing online has as much of an information technology (IT) function now as it does a content function. This essential activity requires tools that can crawl the internet, find you, and fix you. While there are some online tools you can purchase, the digital marketing companies have access to sophisticated programs not available to consumers that do this well. Don't try to do this yourself or have your son's girlfriend who is "really good with technology" try to do this for you. This is a job for your professional digital marketing company. Just as you advise your patients not to do "bathroom surgery," I advise you to leave this to the experts.

Your local search reputation is the "smell test" from prospective patients. They check you out to see if you smell good, bad, or not at all. If your reviews are great and you have a bunch of five-star reviews and recommendations, your practice numbers can soar.

Think about your own behavior. Most of us check reviews before buying products or services—restaurants, concerts, products, services, etc. Inexplicably, we study anonymous reviews from people we don't even know, and we take them very seriously. Armed with this essential information, we collectively make billions of dollars' worth of decisions every day.

Your online reviews are like an advance team that's way out ahead of your office. They guide people back to your online properties and, most importantly, your website. It's essential to establish a habit of generating five-star reviews if you want to be successful.

Your digital marketing company can help you with that. They can set up a system to send your patients a request to review your services after they have an appointment with you. You should use a system like this to get dozens of five-star reviews, but remember that you must provide five-star service to justify those reviews. And if you don't get five-star reviews, have an emergency staff meeting and resolve to get at least one five-star review every day. Put a plan together to make that happen.

There's a right way to get reviews and a wrong way. The right way is to have the reviews posted on a third-party, well-established online platform. The wrong way is to simply post the review or testimonial on your website. While high-quality testimonials on your website are a very good thing—if they're legal in your state—if you have dozens or hundreds on your own site rather than directing your patients to review you on the online platforms, it's an incredible waste of goodwill. Yes, those web testimonials will be great for SEO, and yes, that's a good thing, but the most important places for your patients to say great things about you is on all potential online review sites. If your marketing company recommends that you only post reviews on your own website, walk away. It's a waste of a precious and valuable resource and that company is incompetent.

> I STILL BELIEVE THAT THE SINGLE BEST WAY TO GET GREAT REVIEWS FROM YOUR PATIENTS IS SIMPLE AND EASY. JUST ASK THEM.

I still believe that the best way to get great reviews from your patients is simple and easy. Just ask them. Ask, and ye shall receive. Don't ask, and ye shall be like everyone else with very few or mostly negative reviews. You can and should average one five-star online review per week. That should be your goal because it's achievable. Dr. Peter Wishnie's office in Piscataway, New Jersey has a goal of one five-star review per day, and they often achieve this. To be sure, you can't get great reviews if you don't provide five-star service (and Dr. Wishnie's team certainly does), but you surely won't get them if you don't ask. Here's how to do it in an easy three-step process:

Step I: The best time to get a review or testimonial is when the patient says, "Thank you." When they do, answer, "You're welcome! You know, if all my patients were as delightful as you, I'd be a happier doctor! Would you please let all your friends (the ones like you, not your grumpy friends) know that we'd love to help them if they have any problems? In fact, would you be willing to review us online? Do you know how to do that?" If the patient says yes, then the doctor says "Great! Thank you! Here's a card that gives you the instructions you need to do it." Hand them the card, then make a note in their chart that they received it. And thank them again.

I've got some bad news for you. At this point, most people won't take the time to review you even though they agreed to. They, too, have very busy and complex lives, and this takes some time and thought to accomplish. So, we now move to step two.

Step 2: When the patient checks out, the staff member should see the note stating that they agreed to give a review and say, "I see that you are going to review us online! Thank you so much. We love it when our patients do that! Did the doctor give you the card that tells you how to do it?" Train your staff member to truly show appreciation and express enthusiasm when they communicate this message. I often say that they should act like this patient just invented Christmas. That might be a bit over the top, but you must have a system that includes authentic, happy enthusiasm for their agreement to give you a review.

Guess what? It's still unlikely that they'll review you, even though they're now socially obligated to you and to another very happy person. Their basement is probably flooding as you speak, or something else is going to distract them. That's just how life is. So, on to step three.

Step 3: Your staff member then says, "Good! I'll send you an email right now with all the information and a direct link to the review site.

All you have to do is open the email, click the link, and you can leave that review in no time. Thank you again!" The email is sent immediately.

The email is the clincher. It's so much easier just to click and review. When you follow these steps, you'll probably get two out of ten to follow through on the review. That may sound like a discouraging percentage, and you may see better results, but if you make this a regular habit for you and your staff, your online reviews will climb, and your reception room will be full.

When you implement a review program, you may encounter some resistance from your staff and even from yourself. We don't like to ask people to say nice things about us publicly. Your staff is already very busy, and this additional procedure may be seen as an interruption in their workflow, which is already too time compressed. Persevere with this. Commit this to habit, and you'll be rewarded with a reception room filled with the kinds of patients you want to see.

SOCIAL MEDIA

I think social media is weird. Just weird. It's not even very well understood yet. Sure, it's enabled many wonderful things like closer connections to friends and family. It's allowed businesses to connect to people who want and need their products or services. But it's also been implicated in much that hasn't been good at all.

It's like every other new technology; it's very powerful and amplifies the best and the worst in all of us. In the specific case of doctors who are severely restricted by HIPAA, it isn't very fair, either. But we must take it seriously, and our practices must be online and engaged because millions of people are online every moment of every day. These people need answers to their questions about their health.

It doesn't matter if you personally use or even like social media, your practice must be in the mix, and here's why:

I.   It contributes to your search engine optimization (SEO). The search engines search for new, relevant content they can serve up to their users, and social media posts are part of this search. They provide backlinks to your website and blog and online offers. The more fishing poles you have in the water, the more fish you can catch.

2. It's become such a part of the fabric of our lives that if you don't participate in social media, people who need help will make assumptions about your practice (unfair and inaccurate, but nonetheless real) and the level of care and skill you can provide them. I know—not fair—but important.

It's an essential part of online marketing for medical offices because *she* uses it. Fair or not, women are the primary guardians and caretakers of their family's health. It is she who guides the care for her children and spouse, as well as extended family members such as aged parents. It's not that men aren't engaged, but for the most part, we're marketing to women. And that's great because on social media, women are heavily engaged, interested, and even talented users of social media.

There are some fundamental rules of conduct for professionals who are online and engaged in social media, both personally and professionally. Remember doctor, you're a professional twenty-four hours a day. When you're at the soccer game, you're a doctor. When you're at the grocery store, you're a doctor. When you're at the sports bar—still a doctor. You're a professional, and you should always hold yourself to a higher professional standard.

> THERE ARE SOME VERY IMPORTANT RULES OF CONDUCT FOR PROFESSIONALS WHO ARE ONLINE AND ENGAGED IN SOCIAL MEDIA, BOTH PERSONALLY AND PROFESSIONALLY.

This means you need to keep your political opinions to yourself. No matter what you say, you'll offend half the people who read your posts. That's the nature of politics today. Unless you want to run for office, keep your political opinions offline, especially the political discourse that has become so crude and debased online. Stay away—it's like kryptonite.

If you're a deeply religious person, then be authentic and post inspired religious content that is positive and uplifts the soul from time to time. Just don't overdo it. You're a doctor, not a rabbi, imam, or pastor. They've got their job to do, and you've got yours. Stay focused.

You should post about medical issues and problems that you'd like to treat in your office, and you should do this often. Break these topics into short, one-minute videos or use simple graphics to engage prospective and current patients online. But again, don't overdo it and bore your viewers. Mix it up with interesting and engaged, even inspired, content.

One Top Practices member bought a foot costume online (easy to find, just search for Halloween Foot Costume.) Their marketing staff person is a runner, and he wears the foot costume when he runs in 10ks, 5ks, and walks. He loves this; he's now recognized for it and has dozens of photos across their digital platforms of him in this costume wearing a smile and a big thumbs up as he participates in runs, health fairs, and events in the office. It's fun and funny, and it spices up their social media. Note: If you do this, always be sure the person who is wearing the costume has fun and enjoys this silliness. If not, it can be considered a form of torture!

Post about events that occur in your office and in your community. If you'll be speaking somewhere, make sure that's posted several times before and after the event.

Post uplifting thoughts or original photography. Inspired compassionate messages about our human condition are very appropriate and will help you continue to engage your readers.

Tips to stay healthy and avoid injury also work very well. Fun pictures with your staff and patients are wonderful, too. Always get written permission before you use anyone's image or name on anything you do—it's a legal requirement for patients due to HIPAA.

Your digital marketing company should have powerful tools that allow you to seamlessly link posts across all the major platforms, which allows you to appear to be everywhere at once. The system does all the work for you.

You can't sit out social media. Like it or not, it's part of our lives for the foreseeable future, and if we aren't engaged, we can't contribute to or steer the conversation. Your digital marketing needs to extend across an ever-larger group of platforms, and when it does, the results can be remarkable.

And doctor, you don't need to be the one who does this. Your staff, in coordination with your digital marketing company, can make this happen with very little direct involvement on your part. For the foreseeable future, it's an integral and essential component of any marketing strategy.

But it's still weird.

WE'RE JUST GETTING STARTED

If you speak to most marketers these days, you might be convinced that digital marketing is the entirety of marketing. In fact, most marketing companies are composed of people who know nothing else.

Shhh—here's a secret: We're still marketing to human beings, and human beings still live in an analog world with other humans. Until that changes, *relationships matter.* Experiences matter. Customer service matters. Internet marketing is *only one* marketing pillar. There are still three pillars left for us to discuss, and the one true "silver bullet" in marketing hasn't yet been revealed. Let's leave everyone else behind, gain a competitive advantage that's impossible to overcome, and move on to Pillar Number Two: Referral Marketing.

PROSPERITY TIPS:

- You have a website for one reason, which is to make your practice more profitable. Don't forget that.

- You must work to earn five-star reviews every day.

- Social media is vital and must be engaging, interesting, and designed to drive patients to visit your website or call you.

DISCUSSION QUESTIONS:

- Does your website generate and convert leads for your practice, or have you just checked the "I have a website" box?

- How can you and your staff generate five-star reviews on a consistent basis?

- How are you using social media to advance your internet marketing? How could you improve?

Pillar #2: Referral Marketing

Guess what? Who you know still matters. The three most important words in marketing are nurture, nurture, nurture.

When you first opened your practice, you had lots of time and very few patients, so you did what every professional does—you went out and introduced yourself to anyone and everyone you could. You didn't like it very much. You had no preparation for it, and if you're like many doctors, you weren't well-suited for it.

But everyone in business, and especially every professional, needs solid relationships that send them high-quality referrals. The only way to get those referrals is to ask for them.

When you started your practice, you made those visits, shook hands, and did whatever you could to help you generate good quality referrals from your market. And then at some point, you stopped.

Why did you do that?

You stopped because you didn't like it, not because it didn't work. You also stopped because you ran out of time. Nobody went to podiatry school so they could grow up to sell Girl Scout Cookies, but that's how this feels when you're out there in this face-to-face communication.

You don't want to do this anymore, and you don't have the time to do it, so most of you stopped. You're busy, it's kind of hard, and honestly, who likes to get in the car to go see people? Yet someone must do this job. You need to hire a person, either full- or part-time, to be your shoe-leather marketer. I call this shoe-leather marketing because the person who does this job will wear out the leather on the soles of their shoes. This person will be out in the community meeting people as he or she makes visits to medical and non-medical referral sources on your behalf. You need to have a solid, automated plan to ensure that your referral sources are not only developed, but that they're nurtured, grown, and cared for. That's what this person will do for you.

> YOU NEED TO HAVE A SOLID, AUTOMATIC PLAN IN PLACE TO ENSURE THAT YOUR REFERRAL SOURCES ARE NOT ONLY DEVELOPED, BUT THAT THEY'RE NURTURED, GROWN, AND CARED FOR.

This activity is not *marketing*, however. I define marketing as developing a relationship with someone, when you're not in the same room with them, through a variety of other means. This is different. It is *sales*. Sales is communicating when you're in the room or directly connected to someone.

Above all, hire for personality. This person should be a "ray of sunshine" kind of person who loves to make friends and help people. He or she should also have modern computer skills because they'll need to keep track of their work in a database and produce reports.

Last, this person needs to be mature. By that, I mean they need to be able to work in an unstructured, unsupervised environment because you won't be able to observe their work in the same way you do with your medical assistants. You must be able to trust them.

Here's an ad that Top Practices uses that can help you find your candidates. It was originally written by Dr. Andrew Schneider for his front and back office people. I rewrote it as an ad for a part-time marketing position.

PART-TIME MARKETING POSITION FOR
MEDICAL PRACTICE IN (YOUR TOWN)

- Have you always wanted to work in a small office where you're an integral part of the team?

- Do you want flexible hours?

- Do you love to work with people to help make their experience the best one possible?

- Have you ever visited Disney World and thought "I wish every place was like this!"

If you answered "yes" to all these questions, this job may be for you. We're a busy but small medical practice in [your town.] This position is one of the most important in the practice. It involves representing our practice to the community by visiting medical offices and non-medical businesses. You must have modern computer skills. Also, you must be mature and a real self-starter because much of this job will be done from your home or out in the community.

We will train you how to do this job, but if you need to be told what to do all the time, we're not for you. If you're a person who starts your day with a smile and ends it with a bigger smile, please apply for this position.

To apply, email us. Make sure you spell and write English correctly. The subject line must read: "I'm your new marketing team member." In your email, tell us why you're the best fit to join our team. Let your personality shine.

Also, be sure to send your resume as an attachment to your email. No phone calls—email only. We are ready to hire quickly.

We typically use online job sites like Indeed.com or Craig's List. There's a reason we tell them what subject line to use. It's one of our initial filters. If they don't use that subject line, we don't consider them.

The ad includes even more filters. It says to apply by email. *Email us and make sure you spell and write English correctly.* So, if you get an application in the mail, don't read it. If you get a phone call, don't take it. The only way to apply for this job is through email, and if someone doesn't spell well or write English correctly, they're automatically disqualified.

If they can't follow directions now, they won't follow them later.

In the ad, we also say, ...*tell us why you're the best fit to join our team. Let your personality shine* and *Also, be sure to send your resume as an attachment to your email.* Those things have to happen.

You can also use your own personal network of people as candidates. Your patients are a great source of candidates. Find out how happy they are in their current work. Many of our doctors have found their shoe-leather marketer by opening the opportunity to their patients.

I advise you to get some help when you evaluate the applicants. There's nothing worse than a new hire who doesn't work out. It is painful, it's expensive, and it pushes you further back than you can afford.

This position should be called Director of Community and Patient Relations, not Practice Marketing Person. It shouldn't say anything that identifies them as marketing or sales, and the Director of Community and Patient Relations is a nice, inflated title that doesn't scream sales. It's appropriate because this team member isn't a salesperson; they're a member of a medical team. Their sole focus is to build relationships with other medical practices or companies that can refer you as their trusted specialist in lower extremity problems.

There's only one time when you don't want to use the title Director of Community and Patient Relations, and that's when you advertise for the position. It's a somewhat inflated title, and if you use it when searching for candidates, you may attract people who've held executive marketing positions in the past. They don't want this job, and you don't want to waste your time or theirs. Instead, call the position a Practice Liaison when you advertise. You're looking for someone with retail, sales, meeting planning, or other customer-facing experience. Not marketing. Marketing people have too many bad habits you'd need to break, and it can be frustrating and difficult. Remember, you're primarily hiring for personality.

When I train our own new shoe-leather marketers, I tell them that when they begin to develop referral relationships, the initial goal isn't to get referrals. The goal is to make friends and help people. If the goal for the day is to visit all kinds of businesses and medical offices to make friends and help people, there's a lot less pressure. When the goal is to "get referrals," it's too intense, and it makes people act weird and talk funny—things they wouldn't do if they weren't so worked up and nervous. But if they're there to say "hi" and make friends, there's no pressure, and everyone's a lot more comfortable.

As you start making your visits, you'll need to develop a database to keep track of the medical and non-medical referral sources you've visited. Divide them into groups: A's, B's, C's, and D's.

A's are people who you're already in a referral relationship with.

B's are individuals and businesses that aren't yet a referral source but have the potential to become one.

C's are those with whom you haven't yet made a strong connection. Because something's not working, you might want to postpone seeing them again until the next quarter. Perhaps there will be a different person involved in the future or circumstances might change, but right now you're not making any progress with them.

D's are people who won't refer anyone to you, no matter what. They might already be in a referral relationship with someone else, or they practice in a group and will never be able to send you new patients. For whatever reason, you realize that you won't get referrals from this source, so there's no reason to return.

You must create this list because this legacy information should reside *in the practice*. You want to preserve everything that's been done to connect and where you stand with each one of your referral sources. And when there's a new Director of Community and Patient Relations, they'll be able to pick up where the former person left off, jump right in, and hit the ground running.

The key to success is to regularly visit a high number of potential referral sources. I like to check in with my podiatrist clients and ask them, "Have you been working on your referral relationships?"

They'll say "Yes, we are."

I then ask, "How many have you seen?" I often hear numbers like twenty-five or thirty for the month. The rule of thumb is that for every ten potential referral sources you see, you'll only develop a good referral relationship with about 10 percent.

THE RULE OF THUMB IS THAT FOR EVERY TEN POTENTIAL REFERRAL SOURCES YOU SEE, YOU'LL ONLY DEVELOP A GOOD REFERRAL RELATIONSHIP WITH ABOUT 10 PERCENT.

So, if you visit only twenty or twenty-five, then you can expect one or two potential referral sources to come from that effort. But if you extend your list to three hundred—even upwards of five hundred—you now can expect thirty to fifty good quality, regular referral sources over time.

Think about what that means in potential for your practice. If you can increase the number of referrals, and they're quality patients, the results could be dramatic. That's why this is such a critical component of a good marketing plan. You must stay focused and active, regardless of how difficult it is.

The only way to manage this list is to take the A, B, C, D nomenclature and organize your visits in that way. You'll see your A's regularly, sometimes weekly, because they already send people to you. It's a good business decision and investment of your time. Visit your B's at least once a month, visit your C's quarterly, and never go back to your D's.

Expand your list beyond primary care physicians. Visit OB-GYNs, pediatricians, rheumatologists, endocrinologists, cardiologists, and more. And there's an almost endless number of non-medical businesses around you that can refer people to you like gyms, coaches, senior centers, nail salons, and shoe stores.

Don't be discouraged that about one out of ten will be too busy, too distracted, or just not interested. Your goal is to find those diamonds in the rough that you can polish and turn into something spectacular for your business. That's how you approach this job.

On the first visit, you're just out to say hi and drop off your business card. You're there to make an initial first impression. Respect their time. Don't be there to sell; instead, simply try to help them. Start identifying your A's, B's, C's, and D's, and then go back to see the ones who could be valuable to you.

Don't rush this process. It's like dating; you take it one step at a time, or you'll scare them off.

I'm the happiest married man I know. There are others like me, to be sure, but I don't know anyone more delighted to be married than I am. When I met Diane, she was my co-worker, and I liked her a lot. I didn't, however, look at her and say, "You're great; let's get married!" She would've looked at me—believe me—and said, "You're creepy. Keep your distance." Instead, I got my coffee when she did, I went to lunch with her, and eventually, after several dates, I asked her to marry me, and she said yes.

You're there to date these referral sources, and it'll take time before you can start asking for and getting referrals. Be patient.

So, what can you do in the meantime?

Candy.

One of the most effective marketing tools ever developed since the time of cavemen is the M&M prescription bottle program developed by Dr. Andrew Schneider.

When you visit your current referral sources or potential referral sources, bring prescription bottles filled with M&Ms as a fun leave-behind. (You should have some filled with sugar-free mints for diabetic staff members.) You can print labels for them that might say:

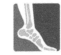

Hollis Foot and Ankle
1555 Arbor Street
Las Vegas, NV 89138
1-888-555-5555

Rx: 8885555555   DR. STUART B. HOLLIS
Take two (2) tablets every time you need to relieve stress
from daily office activities
Qty: We didn't actually count them
Refills: UNLIMITED! Just call us for more

When you show up, find out how many people work in the practice so you can give everyone in the office their own prescription for the M&M stress reduction program.

It's a simple idea and, initially, you might be resistant to doing it. But I'm here to tell you that this is brilliant. It's the best ice breaker ever invented, and it creates excitement (yes, genuine excitement) for your return visits because you bring a big bag of M&Ms and refill everyone's prescription.

You want to be known as the M&M foot guy or the M&M foot lady.

Another great reason to return to the office is to hand-deliver thank-you notes for the patients you've treated that they referred to you. You can also drop off copies of your patient newsletter for everyone in the office. These office workers are people, too, and if your newsletter is interesting, they'll read it.

The members of Top Practices have created dozens of creative, often holiday-themed, leave-behinds. You can do this, too, with a little imagination. It's fun, and it builds those relationships that are so important to your practice.

On about the second or third visit, when it seems appropriate, you can hand out referral pads that make it easier for the doctors to refer to you. All the information they need to easily refer to you should also be on a laminated card that you give to them.

Here's another idea: on the Monday before Thanksgiving, go to your top five or ten referral sources and deliver pumpkin pies with a note that says, "Thank you so much for the trust you place in our practice. Please enjoy this." You'll be the only practice, the only trusted partner, that shows up to their office and makes everybody's Thanksgiving easier through the gift of pumpkin pies.

I want to be clear about this—bring *everyone* who works in the office a pie. If they have twenty people, bring twenty pies. This will blow them out of the water. In my opinion, Costco has the best pumpkin pies, and the price is right, so buy them by the truckload. If you do this annually, you'll start to get calls asking if you plan to do it again this year because they've begun to count on it. It's great!

Don't send holiday cards or treats; you'll get lost in the rush. Think about your own office. How many Harry and David Tower of Treats can you get before you have no idea who sent you what? Send Thanksgiving cards instead. You have the stage all to yourself at that time of year, and it's appreciated.

And on the Fourth of July, do it all over again with apple pies.

Each month, you'll want to arrange Lunch and Learns at their office so you can come in and meet with the doctors and the staff. But don't call them "Lunch and Learns." That term has dropped out of favor. Just arrange to stop by their office with food to share some information with the doctors and staff.

I always say, "Very little learn and lots of lunch." You want to let them know about some of the things that you do in your practice that they aren't aware of. Most people, even other medical professionals, don't have any idea of the extent to which podiatrists can care for their patients. Remember, you can only book Lunch and Learns after you've earned the right to ask for them by building the relationship. It's part of the dating relationship. Just like Rem and Diane.

This is the hardest, has the longest time frame, and is the toughest of all the marketing pillars that we do, but it's also one of the most rewarding. And it's one of the greatest things you can do to build your practice.

Confirm your resolve to get great at this. Remember, referrals will come to you if you have the mindset that they should come to you. They should flow to you in a tsunami, a giant wave, because it's the right thing to do. Expect referrals, don't hope for them. And when you do this, they will be yours.

PROSPERITY TIPS:

- Nurture your referral sources, and they'll reward you for it.

- Hire a "ray of sunshine" person who's responsible for making referral visits and building strong relationships.

- Start doing this now and keep it up until the day you retire.

DISCUSSION QUESTIONS:

- What are you doing to nurture your relationships with your referral sources? How can you improve?

- How can you find the perfect person to handle your shoe-leather marketing? Could it be someone you already know, like one of your patients?

- How accessible and usable is your list of referral sources? How are you tracking this activity? Name some ways you can improve.

Pillar #3: Internal Marketing

The most critical asset in your practice, other than yourself and your well-trained staff, is your list. This is the real secret to medical practice marketing. It's all about your list.

Once again, I must tell you that the three most important words in marketing are nurture, nurture, nurture. People are busy and distracted. They only have enough time to focus on their own worries and concerns. They aren't interested in you or where you went to school. Quick questions: Where did your dentist go to school? How much extra training do they have? What are their clinical qualifications? Do they write for their profession? Are they lecturers? You don't know the answer to any of these questions, right? And, in truth, you don't care. You go to them because the hygienist is gentle with you and the doctor seems fine enough. The bar is very low here. We figure if they aren't in jail, they must be okay.

I hate to break this to you, but nobody cares about you, either. Your mother doesn't care as much as she used to, and your dog might bite you if you stopped feeding her. Just like you don't care about your dentist's qualifications, nobody cares about yours.

Sorry.

I know you worked hard to get them, and it's a tremendous achievement that gives you the right to hold your license and heal people. The problem is that this big, distracted world we live in just doesn't care.

The good news is that we can get people's attention if we focus on what *they* worry about. Things like, "I woke up this morning, stepped out of bed, and had sharp stabbing pains in my heels! What's up with that?" Or, "My father's wound on his lower leg is worse. Why can't we get it to heal?"

People say it's a big, cruel, nasty world out there. That's not been my experience. I think most people I meet are rather nice and aren't trying to hurt me or anyone else. I do know, however, that it's a very distracted world we live in, and it's very easy to be ignored, especially when you're marketing.

Even when we do get their attention, it's often short lived. That's why we make offers of information that they can request so we can send them this useful information and place them into our marketing database. We then continue to speak to them and convince them to come to see us for help. Nurture, nurture, nurture that relationship.

Which brings me to your database.

The number one asset in your practice, other than yourself and your well-trained staff, is your list of people who know you, like you, and trust you. I'll go into more detail about this list, but first I want you to know that this list is the most important component of all your marketing efforts because everything you do, everything you talk about, work on, think of, implement, and innovate is designed to support this marketing pillar.

> THE NUMBER ONE ASSET IN YOUR PRACTICE, OTHER THAN YOURSELF AND YOUR WELL-TRAINED STAFF, IS YOUR LIST OF PEOPLE WHO KNOW YOU, LIKE YOU, AND TRUST YOU.

To understand and then execute well in this pillar is the key. This is the silver bullet in marketing.

A word about silver bullets: A silver bullet refers to an action which offers *an immediate* solution to a problem—a solution that's often magical. But in reality, there's no such thing as a silver bullet that magically solves problems. In our case, it simply means that using your list or database effectively is the central strategy that all your other marketing strategies serve. It isn't magic, but if you appreciate its importance, you'll understand the most critical marketing principle in existence. And you'll never lack for high-quality patients. It's a secret that only the successful understand.

To build and then use this list is the reason we market on the web. It's the reason we market through referrals. It's the reason that we market externally. The foundations that we've built and the tools we use are all designed for one purpose and one purpose only—to help you build an ever-growing list of people who know, like, and trust you because you help them sleep more easily at night.

Your list (or database) is composed of these parts:

- Active patients
- Inactive patients
- Really inactive patients
- Medical and non-medical referral sources
- Everyone who's requested any information from you

It's a database of prospective patients, active patients, referral sources, or potential referral sources that is well organized and continually updated. This list must reside in a database designed for easy use.

Don't use an Excel spreadsheet. You can try, but you won't get very far. In the beginning, if you're on a shoestring budget and you just want to try to figure out how to bootstrap this, an Excel spreadsheet is better than nothing. But it will never scale and will never allow you to manage or accomplish the marketing efforts you need to do with ease.

It's essential that your database is designed for this purpose. This kind of system is called a Customer Relationship Management program or CRM. It's not your EMR (electronic medical records), and it's not your billing software. Those are not designed for this kind of customer or patient contact.

DATABASE: YOUR CUSTOMER RELATIONSHIP MANAGEMENT PROGRAM

The central component of your CRM program is a *contact manager*. This is the actual database in which you store all the information about everyone in your list, including their diagnosis codes or treatment codes. Remember to be compliant with all HIPAA requirements when working with this data. All the information needs to be resident in your database so you can work with it later.

The second major component is what I call the *library*. Think of this library as a building in which there are many shelves and many folders where you can put any kind of book, any kind of paper. Anything that you can think of, you can put in this library. You populate this library with the types of documents you use to communicate with your patients.

Anything you've ever sent out to patients at any time (like letters, emails, videos, documents, handouts, infographics, etc.) should be stored in this library so you know where to find them when you need them. The only exception is out-of-date information, which should be regularly removed. Instead of trying to find the letter that you used two years ago and going to your computer looking under your file structure and doing the usual, *Well, where would I have thought to put that?* It all resides right here in a very organized place called your library.

When your marketing or informational documents are in your library, you can use them in a simple yet powerful way through *campaigns*. Now, the word "campaign" can sometimes be confusing because you can think about a marketing campaign in a variety of ways. In this particular circumstance, what I mean is a sequential communication program or campaign that allows you, over time, to communicate with a specific niche inside your marketing database about whatever topic you wish.

For instance, you can design a campaign for people who have requested information. When someone requests information from you, they're entered into your marketing database and are put into a new patient conversion campaign. And conversion means that you convert them from a prospective patient into a current patient, an active patient. And that campaign is defined inside a marketing database that's set up for this kind of communication.

A new patient conversion campaign is designed to, over time, convert prospective patients into active patients. But you can also market to a niche inside your patient base, such as your diabetic patients. Further, you can establish a reactivation campaign for diabetic patients who haven't been in to see you for a year. Because all the patient information is stored in your database, you know when it's time to re-contact these people. It is easy to use a CRM to automate this strategy. Doing it without this is impossible.

The number of campaigns that you can set up is endless, but I recommend that you start with one or two. One should be designed to convert prospective patients into current patients, and one should be designed to help you reactivate inactive patients, such as your diabetics or people who've been prescribed orthotics, as two examples.

As you move forward with your program, you may decide to layer more and more concurrent campaigns inside your database. Some of our practices have over fifty separate campaigns that run at any given time.

When you first start, just get good at communicating with your patients.

You've certainly been exposed to some famous marketing campaigns, and if you're my age, you can probably remember—in order—the ingredients in a Big Mac® from McDonalds® because their commercials taught us to sing it. And at the time of this writing, the slogan, *"Fifteen minutes can save you 15 percent or more on your car insurance."* is quite popular. GEICO spends hundreds of millions of dollars across all media to ensure that we know this. They spend an exorbitant amount because they knew they had to spice things up because GEICO stands for Government Employees Insurance Company. How boring is that!

MY TREE GUY

A few years ago, my "tree guy" told me he might want a divorce. I'm not kidding.

Diane and I used to live in Pennsylvania (Penn's Woods is the translation) and, believe me, we had trees, a lot of trees, in our yard. We had all kinds of trees, such as evergreens, deciduous conifers, Japanese maples, Cryptomeria that were over eighty feet tall, cherry trees, and in the front yard, two very large sugar maples.

It all started with the sugar maples.

The sugar maples were big, mature trees, and we should've had them trimmed a long time before because they obscured the view of the house from the street. These big maple trees and their lack of curb appeal started to bother Diane, so I called a neighbor who worked with a company that did landscaping. I asked him if his crew would trim our trees back hard.

"Sure!" he said, and then he took months to show up.

I had to bug him multiple times and rather than show up, he just apologized for not showing up. But, in time, his guys finally came, and they did a great job. It was obvious that the trees had been trimmed.

That's what started the trouble.

One crisp, spring morning, I heard our dog barking. She was going nuts like she does when anyone gets within fifty yards of our house. I looked out the window and saw my tree guy spraying the stuff that's supposed to keep my trees healthy. *Good!* I thought. *I need to tell him that the guys who trimmed my trees told me that the cherry trees have scale and need to be sprayed.*

So, I went outside, and my tree guy stared hard at me while I told him about the scale.

When I finished, he cocked his head back and said in a quiet and slow voice, "I see you had your trees trimmed."

"Yes," I said. "That's how I know about the scale."

Continuing to glare, he said, "I'm trying to decide if I'm going to divorce you." I had no idea what he meant.

He continued, "I think I might have to divorce you. I trim trees, you know." Then it dawned on me that he was mad because someone else had trimmed my trees.

"I didn't remember that."

"C'mon, Rem," he said, "when I came out here the first time (over five years ago, by the way), I brought our truck with the bucket lift!" Which, I now know, in tree-guy speak means *I trim trees.* Oops.

"Well, I'll remember that and will call you next time," I said.

Here's the thing—it wasn't my fault. Of course, he hadn't been coached by a marketing expert about the fact that he was responsible for the confusion, so I didn't say anything to him, but I will share the lesson with you. Was it my fault that I didn't remember that he trims trees? The answer is no. That was his responsibility.

The odd thing was that I didn't want the other guys to trim my trees again. It took way too much of my time to get them there. Excellent job, but I needed much better customer service.

Here's the point: It wasn't my job to remember all the services he provides. It was *his* job to continually remind me. It was *his* job to protect and nurture our relationship to ensure and protect his pipeline of future business from dozens of his satisfied customers and from me. To me, he'd become the guy who just sprayed stuff on my trees. Because he allowed that to happen.

Are you making the same mistake with your patients?

What would've happened if he'd sent me a newsletter in February that said any of the following?

You should expect the following things to happen soon in your yard as the winter winds down....

- **The first trees to break their buds are... followed by....**

- **We will visit you soon for these treatments; here is why we do that...**

- **Right now is the optimal time to trim your trees, and we get very busy. Call us now at [phone number] to get your appointment lined up. Call ASAP because we get booked fast, and it might take us longer to get to you.**

I would have read that thing cover to cover. I love stuff like that! I always wondered what the plants in my yard even were. You know what would've happened? I would have canceled the other crew and booked my tree guy. Guaranteed, I would've done that. But he blew it. Big time. And then he lectured me for his lack of marketing.

How guilty are you?

How many times have you found out that your patient had someone else do their surgery because they didn't know you could do it for them? How many patients have you put in a box like the one I put my tree guy in? *Just the guy who sprays my trees. Just the doctor who trims my toenails or helped me with my sprain. I need to see a surgeon for my surgery.* What? Have you ever found yourself muttering something like, "But I parked my truck with a bucket out front!"

NURTURE, NURTURE, NURTURE

With a CRM system, it's easy to stay in touch with your patients. Here are several essential activities you must use to keep in touch with and nurture your relationship with your patients.

Monthly Newsletter:

I realize that monthly newsletters are one of the oldest ideas when it comes to marketing. That's not just true in the marketing of podiatry practices or medical practices or almost every business that there is. In my own business, and in every business that I know, the paper and electronic newsletters we send to our list are one of the most valuable and lucrative marketing programs we could institute. In fact, it's why we spend so much time on web-based marketing, on external marketing. We want to build the list so we can send them information every month.

Yes, your newsletter can be very effective. I can hear some of you say you've used them in the past, and they aren't very effective. And I will submit to you that you most likely sent out what almost everyone sends out—a boring newsletter.

BORING NEWSLETTERS ACCOMPLISH ONE THING: THEY DRAIN YOUR PRACTICE OF MONEY.

Boring newsletters accomplish one thing: they drain your practice of money. But newsletters that aren't boring, that engage and have information that patients are interested in and want to read are essential to your practice growth and need to be built and sustained. You need to nurture your relationship, or they'll quickly forget your name. Remember my tree guy?

Always lead with an article on what condition you'd like to treat the most, like heel pain, because that's what people are going to see first. Promote any of your information pieces, your books, or specials you might offer on new products. You can target segments of your list when you have a marketing database. Say, for instance, you're going to implement a new laser program, a new heel pain program, or even vascular tests. Your database can identify the exact patients you should contact.

Postcards and Email:
Other ways to communicate with those in your database include postcards that promote certain events and products, pertaining to problems that people have during particular seasons. Large format postcards look great and are a cost-effective way to communicate to the niches inside your database. For instance, you can use recall and reactivation campaigns for your diabetic patients, your diabetic shoe programs, your orthotic programs, and for seasonal issues such as the dangers of flip-flops and the alternative footwear you can provide.

How often can you email your patient base without causing them fatigue? Once a week—if you're smart about how you do it.

One of the emails should be your monthly patient newsletter. One should be a video testimonial of a happy patient (if your state allows testimonials). One should be about a procedure such as in-grown toenails, for example, and another about something unrelated to podiatry such as information about a summer concert series or even inspirational topics. If you vary it, and it's interesting and engaging, your patients will read it, feel nurtured, and refer or reactivate in much higher numbers.

It's the "secret sauce" in your marketing mix.

Birthday and Holiday Cards:
Don't forget birthday cards. Some practices still don't send birthday cards to people on their birthdays. It's so effortless. Just collect that information and record it as one of the fields in your database. Send out birthday cards weekly and use colored ink to have every single member of the practice sign them to make them even more personal.

Think about this: Many people will tell you that, in fact, yours is the only birthday card they ever receive. You'll be thanked and appreciated and talked about just because you remember people on their birthday. Can it mean that much to people? Yes, it can, and it does.

If you're going to send cards to your patient base at other times, don't send traditional holiday cards. We're all bombarded by holiday cards, and we can't keep track of or remember any of them. Most people look at them to make sure who they need to keep on their list for next year so they can send them a card. It's a waste of marketing time and money.

Instead, send out Thanksgiving cards. Thanksgiving is a wonderful holiday that everybody is in favor of and supports. And when you do this, yours will probably be the only card they get on Thanksgiving. It's a great way to stay connected.

Remember the pie idea we talked about earlier? Just like you do with your referral sources, invite your patients to come in and pick up a pumpkin pie at Thanksgiving or an apple pie the week of the fourth of July. First come, first served, but all are welcome! It's a beautiful way to nurture and harvest this incredible asset called your database.

Obsess about how you use, nurture, communicate to, and care for that list. Successful practices, successful businesses, successful companies, political parties, and winning campaigns have all cultivated and worked this valuable asset. Some of them spend thousands, and in some cases, hundreds of thousands of dollars to build these lists. They'll invest this money to build and work their list because they know it's their number one asset.

If you make building and using your list your ultimate marketing goal, then you'll be able to roll out anything, fill your treatment rooms to capacity and beyond, and change your mix of patients to be the most optimal and preferable for you. You'll build the practice you want, not the practice that just walks in the door.

Experiential Marketing:
What do your patients experience when they interact with your practice? Each and every patient experience should be well thought out and should be congruent with your beliefs, your character, and your brand.

It begins before they arrive at the office and continues while they're there and even after they leave the office.

The first interaction that many of your patients will experience is through your marketing, so all of it—everything on your website—needs to be current, accurate, and consistent.

The next way they may interact with you is over the phone. Be sure your phone is answered well. You spend an enormous amount of time, effort, money, thought, and care to get that phone to ring, and in many cases, that could be where you lose an opportunity with a prospective patient, or even in some cases, your active patients.

> THE FIRST INTERACTION THAT MANY OF YOUR PATIENTS WILL EXPERIENCE IS THROUGH YOUR MARKETING, SO ALL OF IT—EVERYTHING ON YOUR WEBSITE—NEEDS TO BE CURRENT, ACCURATE, AND CONSISTENT.

My favorite way to answer the phone is, "Welcome to [Your Practice]." The word welcome is a surprise in this instance. It's fresh, and it has a wonderful sound to it. (It's much better than what Alexander Graham Bell proposed as the way we answer the phone, which was "Ahoy!") Answering the phone with welcome is an example of what I call a "pattern interrupt." The caller will know that you're different from the moment the phone is answered. They'll see that you're welcoming, that you're not like everyone else.

I hate to be the one to break this to you, but no matter how well you think your phones are being answered right now, they're not answered or managed as well as you think they are. The reason I know this is because it's true in every practice, even in the well-managed practices. Unless you pay attention to how your phone is answered and train your people to do it right, it's just another distraction for your busy staff. It's just one more thing they have to deal with. But in reality, it's critical to your practice's health.

Consider having your practice mystery shopped. Mystery shopping is when someone contacts your office via phone, poses as a patient, and experiences the entire process. That's how you'll find out whether it's being done the way you want. Mystery shopping creates an excellent opportunity for you to train your staff to take care of this crucial moment when you can put your best foot forward.

This should go without saying, but your office must be clean. Sparkling. Fresh and Inviting. Try this: no matter how you usually enter your office, try going in through a different door. Use the exact same entrance that your patients use. As you walk up to your office, take a look at everything. Are there cobwebs somewhere? Is there paint that's peeling? How inviting and friendly does the atmosphere seem at your building? Take a look at the signage outside, the signs on your door, and when you go inside, the signs and your logos on your office walls and in your treatment rooms. Are they new and fresh, or have they been faded by the sun?

How inviting and friendly is your reception room? Sit down in it when your patients aren't there. Just walk in, sit, look around, and experience your waiting room. What does the carpet look like? What do the walls look like? Is this an office that communicates a professional, friendly, up-to-date space, a place you want to be? Or is that stain in the carpet from 1962 still there?

You're probably so familiar with your office that you can't really see it anymore. But your patients do. What's the condition of the chairs? What are the magazines like? What kind of information—useful content—is available for your patients to read? Is your waiting room filled with old, thumbed-through magazines that are so uninviting you don't want to pick them up, or do you have crisp, new magazines and useful pamphlets they can enjoy?

Do you have flyers for all your information, including your books and any kinds of programs that you have available? Does the TV have some horrific news on it, or are there good quality video programs that run in a nice loop on your beautiful flat-screen television that shows that you're current and state of the art?

Are all your products neatly displayed, and are they attractive, arranged, and packaged by your staff who knows how they work and how they fit into your protocols?

When your patients arrive, does your staff collect everyone's email address as part of the patient's contact information? You already know that your email list is an essential and critical part of excellent database management. Every person who walks into your door may not have an email address, but well over 95 percent do. And, even then, some of those people may not want to give you their email address because they don't want to get more emails.

When this happens, your staff can remind the patient that you collect email addresses so you can communicate with them in the most effective way possible. It also helps your practice be as "green" as it can. And, from time to time, you'll send some information to help them stay healthier. And oh, by the way, we're your doctors, so we're not only legally bound to keep your information private, but we would never share your email address with anyone else.

Collecting a good, solid, usable email for every patient is critical to good internal database marketing.

The entire patient experience should be as enjoyable as possible and so good it can even get you some buzz (Buzz is when they talk about you to others.) Here's one great way to generate fun buzz about your practice: ice cream or frozen yogurt prescriptions. It's simple, and your patients will love it. Here's how it works:

> COLLECTING A GOOD, SOLID, USABLE EMAIL FOR EVERY PATIENT IS CRITICAL TO GOOD INTERNAL DATABASE MARKETING.

Set up a coupon reimbursement program with a local ice cream parlor or frozen yogurt shop. If they're smart, they'll do this for free because no one comes in to get a free ice cream cone without bringing three or four other people. Any time you're with a patient, look at them, reach in your pocket, and say, "I've got one more prescription I think would be good for you."

Have a little fun when you do this. Go through all the motions of writing a prescription. Sign it, pull it off the pad, and hand it to them.

They'll look at it and say, "This is for ice cream."

And you'll say, "Yeah, I just thought an ice cream might be something you'd like today. Go to this local shop and get an ice cream cone on us."

When they leave your office, not only have you done something that no one's ever done for them before, but when they either get back to work or when they see their friends or family, they'll say, "You won't believe what my podiatrist did for me today!" They'll tell the story of the prescription you wrote, and the listeners are likely to ask, "Hey, do you think he or she could help me? I've got this problem..."

Here are a couple more ideas about giving your patients an engaged, exciting, interesting, and noteworthy experience; that is, something that they would buzz about.

Make sure you call all new patients the night of their first appointment. All the doctors who do this say it takes almost no time because the patients rarely have questions. But they've never experienced this high level of service before with other doctors. It's a personal touch. Of course, you'll also call all surgery patients that night just to make sure they're okay.

Most patients don't enjoy their time in the waiting room, so have your staff offer them little snack boxes that contain simple, healthy snacks. A small refrigerator underneath the reception desk could hold small bottles of water you can give them. These little things make it a pleasant experience and add up to something much larger over time. But beware! When you start something like this, you should continue it because you don't want to disappoint people. They'll remember it, expect it, and sorely miss it if it's absent.

For example, I used to fly out of the Philadelphia airport regularly, and I'd park at Smart Park where they gave me a little roll of Smarties candies when I rolled out to pay my bill. I don't like those, so I switched to All Day Park, which gives me a cool bottle of water as I drive out. And it's such a nice thing. If someone doesn't offer me that water bottle—and it has happened—I ask about it. And if I didn't get it, I'd be super disappointed. It's one of the reasons, as crazy as it may sound, that I park at that specific parking lot even though it's farther away. It has nothing to do with their service or their parking or where the lot is; it's all about that bottle of water.

I've already suggested that you answer your phones by saying, "Welcome." When someone walks into your office, the first thing they should hear is also "Welcome." And when they see *you*, they should hear *you* say, "Welcome, it's great to have you here today." By the time they see you, they'll feel very welcomed and much appreciated for the very special people that they are: your patients, the lifeblood of your practice.

The opportunities to surprise and nurture your patients are almost endless, and their perception of their level of care is just as important to them as the outcomes are. Thoughtful marketing time spent here is an incredible investment in your future success.

PROSPERITY TIPS:

- The most important asset in your practice, other than you and your well-trained staff, is your list.

- Nurture your list by educating your patients at least once per week. It will reward you.

- The customer experience you and your staff provide will determine how fast and how far your practice grows. Focus on making it exceptional.

DISCUSSION QUESTIONS:

- Where do you store your patient contact information? Can you use your current system for marketing, or do you need to upgrade to a CRM?

- Who in your practice is responsible for ensuring that you're marketing to your patients every week through education?

- On a scale of one to ten, how would your patients rate their customer service experience at your office (one being terrible and ten being the best they've ever experienced)?

Pillar #4: External Marketing

The entire purpose for externally marketing your practice is to build your list. This is the most expensive, the most difficult, and the most frustrating of the four pillars. External marketing is the pillar in which the return on your investment is the lowest. So, it begs the question, *Why do it?* You do it because your top goal in marketing your practice is to build your list. As you build your list *and use it*, you'll get the ultimate result you want, which is to see more of the kinds of patients that you want in your practice.

You already know that you can market your practice online (Pillar #1), you can market it to medical and non-medical referral sources near you (Pillar #2). You can market to your own list (Pillar #3), and you can market to the broader community through advertising, sponsorships, broadcast, community involvement, and public speaking (Pillar #4).

When you build your list and make it bigger and more targeted, you have more control and more access to a group of people who'll be much more responsive and will help build your practice. This is how you get double-digit results from your marketing. External marketing is an essential tool to feed that list.

The primary goal of marketing your practice this way is to do one of two things: either get new appointments immediately or get leads that convert into appointments and patients at a later date.

THE PRIMARY GOAL OF MARKETING YOUR PRACTICE THIS WAY IS TO DO ONE OF TWO THINGS: EITHER GET NEW APPOINTMENTS IMMEDIATELY OR GET LEADS THAT CONVERT INTO APPOINTMENTS AND PATIENTS AT A LATER DATE.

The hardest and most expensive place to market is where people are when they're not looking for information or help. And thousands of them don't even have a problem you can solve. So, again, we need to ask the question, Why market here at all? The answer is because of the sheer volume of people.

If you use the channels and techniques discussed in this module effectively, you can reduce your costs and increase the number of new patients and new leads in a way that you can't accomplish anywhere else. When this works, it's a wonderful thing. Although all four of the pillars are equal in terms of their importance, I suggest that you make sure you execute the other three pillars effectively and optimally before you spend much time on this one. This pillar is about the long view. It will take time for it to work, but when it does, it will drive all the other pillars.

Remember this: you are never branding yourself, or as people often say, "getting your name out there." Not now, not ever. This bears repeating because you'll be tempted to talk about yourself and how you treat your patients like family.

Remember:

- People don't care about you.

- People don't believe anything you say in marketing.

No one wakes up in the morning and says, "I would just love to learn about the local podiatrists in my area today. I wonder if they're board certified. I wonder where they went to school?" That never happens.

And yet, within your reach are hundreds and thousands of people who have problems with their feet and ankles or know someone else who does. And they're intensely interested in what you do. If you can engage them in such a way that you can generate either (a) an

> REMEMBER THIS: YOU ARE NEVER BRANDING YOURSELF, OR AS PEOPLE OFTEN SAY, "GETTING YOUR NAME OUT THERE." NOW NOW, NOT EVER.

appointment or (b) a lead (which can lead to a future appointment), then you can build a list of people who are thinking about foot and ankle problems.

When people are concerned about these problems, they want information about what keeps them up at night. You already know what they think about because they tell you every day in your treatment rooms.

"I'm worried about the bump on the side of my foot that's gotten worse."

"I'm really concerned about the wound on my dad's leg that won't heal, no matter what the doctor tries to do to help him."

The single, most powerful thing you can offer them is the information they want. Websites accomplish this task well, but what you can't get when you put this information online are the names and emails of the people who browse your site. You need a strategy to collect that information. Here it is:

We ask them.

It's that simple. We ask them to give us their name and a good email address. In some cases, we might even ask for their postal address or phone number. You might think that nobody will give out their name and email anymore.

You would be wrong about that.

People hand over high-quality information to all kinds of professionals and companies every day. The simple way you can do this is to offer them something they want that's very easy to deliver to them at little to no cost.

You can offer them a book. When you produce a book and offer it to anyone who requests it, you'll need to collect information so you can send it to them. It's that simple. Did you know that word *authority* contains the word *author*?

Here's Dr. Craig Thomajan's book on heel pain that we produce for our Top Practices members. It answers the questions that prospective patients ask, such as, "Why do I have sharp stabbing pains in my heels when I step out of bed in the morning? What caused that? How can I end this?"

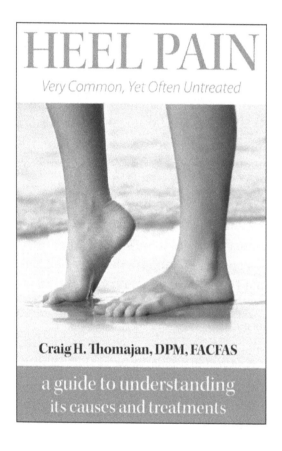

Your ability to make compelling offers is one of the most effective strategies to bring in patients who've expressed an interest in your practice or your services. It all starts with a targeted message that grabs their attention, which is used in social media advertising, emails, websites, videos, and much more.

You can also expand the reach of your offer through ads and messages that direct your prospective patients to take a quiz to learn more about their condition. Adding quizzes helps prospective patients find out more about their heel pain and is key to moving them through the process. Quizzes are fun, quick, and easy, and they significantly increase engagement and interest.

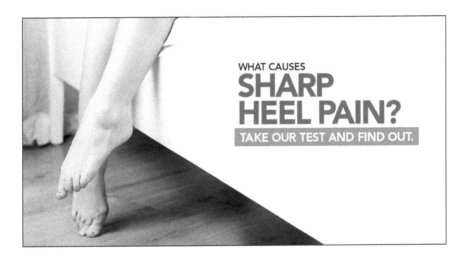

WHAT CAUSES
SHARP HEEL PAIN?
TAKE OUR TEST AND FIND OUT.

We use quizzes that have an accurate etiology, depending on how the patient answers the questions, so they get a result that's consistent with their answers. The patient can then either call your office to make an appointment or they can easily request a copy of your free book, which is instantly delivered to them via email.

Once you have their contact information, present yourself as the authority on the subject (because you are), and then send them follow-up marketing messages to encourage them to make an appointment to get their heel pain under control. You'll continue to market to them until they make that appointment or ask you to stop.

You already know it can take people a long time to "think about it" before they come in to see you. It's human nature. You can't change that, but you can meet them where they are as they worry about their painful problem that only gets worse. When they're finally ready, you'll be the one they call. Don't be surprised if it takes months or even years. That doesn't really matter unless you plan to retire soon. You'll be ready to help the pipeline of your perfect patients that your marketing has delivered to you.

You won't convert your entire city, county, or town, and you don't need to. You only need to convert the people who've raised their hand and requested your book. Market to them. No matter where you practice, there are more than enough feet for you to build a prosperous, profitable, enjoyable practice.

There are no bad markets, only bad marketers.

IS PRINT DEAD?

Print isn't dead yet, but it's dying. When I think about print, what comes to mind are newspapers, shopping guides, penny savers, and women-focused publications. Some people still live in markets where newspapers produce good results, but these are increasingly rare.

Print is frustrating. It takes testing, and the results are variable. Everything requires testing, but print can be expensive to test. When it works well, it's productive and can be worth it. You can test with your local newspapers, and what I mean by testing is that you don't get locked into any kind of a long-term agreement. Make them work for it and test the results. They will push for a long-term contract, and you'll want to negotiate very hard with the salespeople who sell newspaper ads. If they won't bargain with you, walk away. Be very, very hesitant to get into anything that locks you into a contract.

Newspapers are tough to use as an advertising conduit. Much better options are the little shopper guides, pennysavers, merchandisers, fish-wrap kind of things that are tossed in your driveway without you requesting them. They're also in places like restaurants, lobbies, beauty salons, and professional offices. The cost to advertise in these is usually lower than in the newspaper.

One reason for this has to do with circulation. Newspapers have a very large circulation (which is actually shrinking every day), but the pennysavers often have a limited or a regional circulation, so you won't spend as much money to advertise in those. Think about what happens to those publications when they show up at your house. They're picked up, they're dropped on the kitchen counter, and they sit around. Multiple people could potentially read them because the content isn't time critical like it is in a newspaper.

The pennysavers come out every week or two, and they typically last about two weeks in a home. (If they're in my house, they're read at the table by Diane and anyone else who happens to be in the house.) As a result, you'll have a higher return on investment for those than you would for the newspaper—unless you have a fabulous newspaper. Which leads us to the sweet spot: women-focused publications.

In Lancaster County, Pennsylvania, there's a publication called *Lancaster County Woman.* It has a circulation of 75,000 copies, and it's delivered to every driveway. Every two months, they publish this thing that contains articles alongside ads. The focus is on health, fashion, salons, aesthetic surgery, and more. Since women are generally responsible for making these kinds of decisions for themselves and their family, this is an excellent way to reach them.

Beware: You'll be tempted to advertise in the high-end, glossy, beautiful color publications that are distributed in more affluent markets or neighborhoods with a higher socio-economic index. But I have to tell you, we've found these readers to be almost non-responsive. The nicer the publication, the lower the return that you'll see. I don't know why this is, but I know that it's true. At the most, try one ad and see if you get any response at all.

TV AND RADIO

What about broadcasting on television and radio?

> IN MY OPINION, TELEVISION IS A GREAT ADVERTISING MEDIUM, BUT IT'S EVEN BETTER WHEN YOU GET IT FOR FREE.

Very few podiatrists that I know take advantage of television. In my opinion, television is a great advertising medium, but it's even better when you get it for free. Here's how you do that: make friends with the local editors and/or producers at your TV and radio stations. These are the folks who are responsible for health content in their media environment, and they're starved for content. They have deadlines. They have endless waves of deadlines that come at them over and over again. They need good content.

You can find them online. They're there, I guarantee you. Friend them on Facebook. Follow them on Twitter, Instagram, or anywhere they are. Figure out their email address. My email at Top Practices is Rem@TopPractices.com, and it's the same format for everyone in our company. We use first names followed by our domain name because we're a small company. There are no other Rems and no other Dianes, so it's pretty simple. If I worked at a large company, I might be rem.jackson@company.com or rem_jackson or rjackson. Whatever the email convention is for one person, it will be the same format for everyone else, so it's an easy way to figure out people's email addresses.

You'll have to prove to them that you're reliable, you're a good source of information, and you'll provide content that will be helpful to them. Don't ever tell them, "I'd be glad to talk about these topics because I do this and I do that," or, "People need to know this, and we just got this machine that's cool and blah, blah, blah."

They don't care.

They care about what their listeners or viewers are interested in.

You can set Google Alerts for the kinds of keywords that are conditions you treat (e.g., heel pain, plantar fasciitis, fungal toenails, broken toes, broken foot, ankle sprain), and Google will notify you whenever these keywords appear online. What's great about getting these alerts is that celebrities sometimes experience problems with their lower extremities. My classic example is Eli Manning, quarterback for the New York Giants, who had plantar fasciitis. When one of our doctors received a Google alert about it, he immediately contacted his local media editors.

Your message to them could contain something like this:

Tell them that Eli Manning, quarterback of the New York Giants, was diagnosed with plantar fasciitis, otherwise known as heel pain. Tell them what the condition is and what it means to their readers/viewers/listeners. Offer more information that could be useful. Offer to follow up with expert advice on this story and give them your full contact info.

Send press releases to these people, communicate with them and prove that you're reliable, you know what you're doing, and you "get it." Your job is to help them with their agenda, not push your own. It could take a month, six months, a year, or even several years, but once you've developed a relationship and gotten inside the door, you'll become their go-to person. The next thing you know, you're on the radio. You're on the television. You'll be in the newspaper all the time.

If you don't believe me, just take a look at your local papers and take a look at national news. You'll see that they always go back to the same people. The reason they go back isn't that those people have any more expertise or knowledge than anyone else. It's because they're reliable, they're fast, and they're responsive. Don't make journalists or TV and radio producers wait. They operate on very, very strict deadlines.

EVENTS AND PUBLIC SPEAKING

Most people don't enjoy public speaking, and many dread it. If you have the opportunity to address groups in your area, it can be an excellent resource to find new patients if done well. Delivering a talk to groups of diabetics, athletes, or other members of the public is a great idea.

But here's the thing: Remember that when you address the public, you have three goals. The first is to teach and help people be healthier. The second and third goals (I hope you know them by now) are to generate appointments or generate leads for appointments later. In other words, build your list.

Let people know that you've published a book, such as the book *Heel Pain* that you can purchase from Top Practices, and give them an easy way to request a copy. Bring a support person with you, and two-thirds of the way through your talk, ask that person to pass out one-page flyers where they can request your book. Give them time to fill out the forms and pass them back in. If your CRM permits, you can ask them to send a text to a specific number to request a copy of your book.

When you do that, if you speak to forty people, you won't just talk to forty people who won't remember your name five minutes after they hear it, even if they're interested in what you have to say. You will instead leave with thirty, twenty, fifteen—even if it's just ten—of those people's information in your database. If there are forty people and ten requested your book, that's great! Because if thirty people heard you speak and aren't interested enough in what you had to say to request a copy of your free book, then you don't want them in your database. There's no way that they'll convert into a new patient. They don't have a problem you can solve right now. But when you find ten or fifteen people who do have a concern or worry, they're a valuable addition to your list.

Now you can begin to "speak" to those people over the weeks and months ahead to convert them into patients. This is a beautiful way to build your list of prospective patients, and over time, convert them into new patients.

SPONSORING EVENTS

You can find many opportunities to be involved in sponsoring events. Some of them are useful, and some aren't. Let's examine one that's very common and perfectly suited to podiatrists: local races and walks.

When you sponsor an event, they'll put your name on the banner, event program, T-shirts, and tote bags. They'll thank you on the website, and you can have a booth to hand out things while you're there. Fine. In my opinion, those are the least valuable parts of a sponsorship deal because, on the day of the event, people are absorbed *in the event* itself. They don't really want to talk to you.

Think about your own experience when you go to a health fair or any kind of an exhibition. You walk around, and you grab tons of things. When you leave, you've got a bag full of stuff that you don't really care about. There might be one or two things that grabbed your attention and made you think; *I'm going to check into that.* But as a rule, ninety percent of what you collected will land in a pile until you throw it away.

It's very costly for those event sponsors. They've spent time and money to produce those things and engage you, and you ultimately ignore them.

Very difficult.

When people are at a race or an event, they're caught up in the moment and won't remember you or anything about any of that stuff you gave them.

What's most important in sponsorship is what happens *before* and *after* the event. This is your time. Since practically no one else engages with the participants then, you'll have the field to yourself. If you work with a race event or sponsor a little league team, they'll probably put your name on the back of their shirts. But there's also a message you want to deliver. I'd say it like this:

> *One thing that's very important to understand about Dr. Jones is that he has a very deep commitment to ensuring that everyone in our region who's concerned about their feet and their ankles has the information they need so they can make informed choices about their health.*
>
> *We're dedicated to education. Before the event, we want to work with you to help teach and guide the runners who will participate. We want to ensure they have the information they need to take optimal care of their feet and ankles so they can run this race injury and disease-free. We'll contribute content for your website and social media to help people train and prepare for this race."*

Engage the event planners from an educational standpoint. This can be fun because your message isn't, "We'd like some exposure before the event" or, "We want you to point people to our website." Of course, they'll ask how much you're willing to pay for that, and you can let them know that you're "committed to providing free information to anyone that wants it."

Turn it around, and hand something to people. Give them help and information. Tell them you've published a book such as the book *Running* that Top Practices can produce for you and give a free copy to everyone who runs in the event. Give them the promotional copy and links to your offer. Ask them to email it to the participants and include it in their social media broadcasts.

Say that you want to congratulate their participants on running the race and achieving their goals and want to make sure that they're able to do this for the rest of their life both injury and disease-free.

Always remember that when you give presentations or sponsor events, your goal is to generate appointments and leads. Never, ever, ever forget your goals!

ALWAYS REMEMBER THAT WHEN YOU GIVE PRESENTATIONS OR SPONSOR EVENTS, YOUR GOAL IS TO GENERATE APPOINTMENTS AND LEADS. NEVER, EVER, EVER FORGET YOUR GOALS!

You can be as creative with this as your imagination allows. Our members are routinely generating new and imaginative ways to market externally. Quite possibly my favorite example of creativity comes from the team of Dr. Jane Graebner from Delaware, Ohio. Her staff worked with the city of Delaware to have every August 30th declared "Be Kind Day." On the inaugural day, they invited local leaders, the press, and other professionals and businesses to their office for the first celebration of "Be Kind Day." This is an example of how giving back to their community in such a positive way has allowed them to forge relationships with influencers and extend their community outreach with no overt marketing messaging. Simply making friends and helping people.

Nurture, nurture, nurture.

External marketing, Pillar #4, is not the easiest pillar, and it can be the most expensive one if you're not careful. But when you're prepared with good strategies, tools, and offers, you can tap into this bountiful resource to build your list and achieve your marketing goals.

I HAVE SOME GOOD NEWS!

We're finished discussing the Four Pillars. I often think of podiatry practice marketing as a climb up a steep cliff. You've now made it to the top of that cliff, and as you stand on this new higher ground, you can see that there aren't any more cliffs to climb. There aren't any higher levels you need to understand. This is it. This is great practice marketing. From this point on, everything comes down to execution and mindset. You'll just have to get great at this.

Think about it like this: Remember the first time you held a scalpel and made the initial incision in another person's body? That was a momentous occasion for you, right? Now you've done it so often that it's just another Friday morning for you. You practiced, and you achieved mastery. That same journey is before you, but this time, you're armed with this information. It will take time and commitment, but you can turn your practice marketing into the equivalent of "Friday morning."

But you aren't there yet. There's still the matter of your management and your mindset.

PROSPERITY TIPS:

- Remember that no one cares about you. They only care about and focus on their own worries and concerns. Market to that.

- Offer high-quality information that answers the question, "What's keeping them up at night?"

- Make sure you have the first three pillars in excellent condition before you spend money on advertising and sponsorships.

DISCUSSION QUESTIONS:

- What are the key conditions you would like to see in your practice every day?

- What information are you using to build your list? How can you improve?

- Are you ready to advertise or market using broadcast or other advertising venues? How will you catch these leads and convert them?

GOALS

Goals that are not written down are just wishes.

—ANONYMOUS

You've heard that you need to set goals. If you're like I used to be, you nod in agreement and then do nothing to get serious about creating or achieving goals. Maybe it's because you're doing all right without them, or so you think. Most of us have good lives. We have shelter, safety, food, security, and love in our lives. And yet we're unhappy about how much, or what kind of safety, food, security, and love we have. The years go by, and we seem to be stuck in neutral, just happy enough, but not fulfilled. And as is often the case, life comes along, kicks us pretty hard, and asks, "How serious are you about living a successful life as you define it?"

I never wrote down my goals until January 2007, when I started Top Practices. That's when I wrote down my business, personal, financial, health, and fun goals on 3x5 cards. In fact, I always carry those original 3x5 cards with me. I've now met and exceeded almost every one of those goals, and most have been achieved in a very different way than I anticipated when I wrote them.

The list of successful people who attest to the power of written, reviewed, and revised goals is almost endless. If you want to achieve deep success filled with rewards, you must become committed to a process to write down and achieve your goals.

The Top Practices Plan to Achieve Your Goals

The best day to commit to writing down and achieving your goals has passed—it was the day you opened or bought your own practice. The second-best day is today. No matter what time of year it is, get started now and don't stop.

To be clear, start now, but then I want you to consider the summer months to be your time for business development and goal development. Start in late May and finish in early September.

Most people think this is counter-intuitive. Summer is the time to take a break, go on vacation, or just slow down. You should still do all those things in the summer, but if you plan out twelve weeks of goal and business development work, when September comes, you'll be ready to hit the last quarter of the year and all of the next year with a clear vision and plan.

Everyone else will wait and become serious at the end of the year, and most won't get started even then. They'll then tell themselves the big lie—I'll do it over the holiday break—which we've all said but have never done. Then they move on to first-of-the-year resolutions and plans, which don't last long. Before you know it, another year has gone by.

Summer goal work helps you avoid all of that, and you'll feel like a winner on New Year's Eve when you're ready to achieve your goals for the months ahead.

Summer is a twelve-week period, and in the U.S., it unofficially starts on Memorial Day and ends on Labor Day. I do recognize that while we're having winter here, they're having summer in the Southern Hemisphere. For those of you who are "down under," you'll have to make that seasonal adjustment.

As the author Simon Sinek says in his book *Start with Why: How Great Leaders Inspire Everyone to Take Action*, if you don't start out with why, you'll get knocked off your path at some point. Maybe right away, perhaps in a little while, but at some point, the world will conspire against you to knock you off your path. I promise you; it happens to all of us. Even with your big why's.

Pursuing goals isn't easy. I struggle too. People who know me know I have goals for my health and for weight loss. These have always been a challenge for me. I have self-discipline, desire, focus, literally everything I need to achieve these goals, yet I struggle with them.

My "why" for my health goals is very easy to put into specific terms. I want to see my grandchildren graduate from high school or even higher. And things were on track for me and my health goals until I broke my ribs on January 26, 2016—at 8:00 a.m.—and, boy, oh boy, I'll tell you what, talk about a setback for that particular goal. I tried multiple times to go back to my yoga program and to work on my health goals but with no success.

I just stopped—again.

Most of us don't even know why we stop. Why did I get serious in the first place? Why did I fall off? It just seems to happen, and it happens to *all* of us.

As I said, I have a specific and clear vision of my *why* for my health. I imagine this scenario all the time when I think I don't want to work out. I think of Diane twenty-plus years in the future at a grandchild's graduation with our daughters and the rest of our family.

She looks at one of our daughters and says, "You know, your father would have loved this. He would have been so happy to be here."

That makes it real for me. I don't want that to happen. You've got to find one of those "I don't want this" scenarios that works for you. It should give you a gut-check reminder of what your goals mean to you. My imagined scenario would be terrible. I want to be there with my family, loving every second. I don't want to be the guy who didn't make it. Now, if it's in the cards that I don't make it, then so be it. That's fine. I'm at peace with that, but I don't want to help it come about because I like pizza and wine as much as I do.

It's easy to get off track. Business challenges will hit you from time to time. We all get what I call *stink bombs* at least three times a year. For example, your people will quit. Good people quit in your practice, sometimes all at once. Associates will quit. People will betray you. I've seen this often, much more than I could have imagined when I started Top Practices. Institutions will mess with you. Letters will come. Bigger issues will find their way to you like illness, divorce, and much, much more.

Ribs are going to get broken from time to time.

It's not easy to stay focused, and if you don't know your why—your very big why—then you can't remind yourself why you need to accomplish your why—*so I can see my grandkids graduate from high school, God willing. Or I'm doing this so I can have the lifestyle I want and not just to work harder and harder.*

Here are my essential questions to think about as you build your *why* for your business.

Ask yourself these questions:

- What's the purpose of my career?

- Why do I go to work every day?

It can't only be "because I have patients scheduled." It can't be "because I have to make money." There has to be something bigger, something much more important to you. For every goal you work on, you must know the why of that goal. You

FOR EVERY GOAL YOU WORK ON, YOU MUST KNOW THE WHY OF THAT GOAL.

must commit to your *why* for every one of your goals because it's this focus that will make it stick.

As I coach my members, especially those who are in their forties, I find that they begin to question their passion and their purpose because they are just okay. They work hard and have some success, but things have started to feel pretty routine. This happens to almost everyone.

When you know your *why,* it can make all the difference as you navigate this challenge that we all face. Why do you go to work? What are the blessings—the unbelievable blessings that your career has provided you? What does your career make possible? Why do you go to work, and what does it mean to you?

I believe that, at our core, we work to provide for the emotional and financial stability and security of our loved ones and ourselves. Visualize in great detail what that means to you. Otherwise, the endless waves of people and challenges that constitute your daily work can grind your soul into dust. There must be a higher and noble purpose for your work. You must have a *why*.

This has to be personal for you. What do *you* get out of it? This is important because it can't be everybody else who gains from what you do. What do *you* get out of it? What do you think you *should* get out of it? Is there a difference between those two answers? If there's a difference, why do you think that is? What needs to change to reconcile those differences, because if you want to be happy, you have to find a way to solve this problem. Ask yourself this question I learned from Dan Totaro, a therapist who specializes in healthcare professional issues such as addiction, fatigue, and burnout:

"If I keep up things the way they are now, will I be able to sustain this for the next twenty years?"

That's a big question, and it puts a fine point on this important issue. If the answer is "no," (and it is for many of us) then what do you need to change to reconcile these differences? What will you do to make that happen? For you to create vibrant goals that are sustainable, you must know the answer to this question.

What tools will you use to make this happen? Who will you work with to make this happen, and why should they care?

Once you've developed your plan, how will you determine if you get off track? How will you know? Because that's going to be a problem. We all get off track, and we often don't even notice. Suddenly, we're twenty-five pounds heavier, and we didn't notice it happening. That happened to me. So, how do you get back on track?

Start with your *why* because if you don't know why, it will be impossible to get to the how's and the what's that you will focus on to achieve your goals.

Some of you will want to speed this up. You'll say, "I want to move faster." Don't do that. Take your time with this. Be thoughtful and do this well. You'll get a lot more out of it.

The Deceptively Simple Yet Extremely Powerful (DSYEP) Tool to Get Organized

Knowing your *why* is where to start. But how do you get started?

You get organized.

You clear the decks and focus on what you should do, not the endless paralyzing list of what you could do. None of us has unlimited time and energy, and we all have extensive to-do lists. Very few understand the need to create a should-do list and focus on that list and that list alone.

I created my Deceptively Simple, Yet Extremely Powerful (DSYEP) tool to get organized for one reason: self-preservation. The people who work with me think I'm very organized and that I remember everything. While this is somewhat accurate in my business life, it's not how my friends and family see me. They think I'm a nice airhead who rarely knows much (or anything) about what's going on. Whenever Top Practices members make a comment to my daughters about what it must be like to have a father with my organizational skills, they respond, "Do you mean *my* dad?"

My natural set point is to be creative, not organized. Early in my career, I had the self-awareness to realize this, and I used tools to help me achieve the kind of organizational, management, and planning skills I knew I needed. They have served me well.

I created the DSYEP prioritization tool to help me overcome the endless things I knew I should do but never had the time to do. If you hear yourself say, "I just don't have enough time to do the things I know I should do," then this tool is for you. You do have the time. You have the exact same amount of time as every other person you've ever met. A few of us have figured this out, and it's a key to our continued success.

DSYEP

Step I:

Make an appointment with yourself to go to a safe place where you can avoid distractions and interruptions. This could be a library or coffee shop or park, or even an office. Be prepared to spend three hours of quality time to accomplish this goal. Bring your snacks and drinks. Turn off all connections to the outside world—all computers, phones, you name it, in airplane mode or off. No wi-fi. Nothing.

Step 2:

Make a list of everything you have to do. Everything. Hold nothing back; no task is too small to make this list. This includes everything you should be doing for work, for your family, your house, chores—everything. Just get it all down on paper or in a document. Spend a good amount of time on this.

The goal is to get it out of your head and into this vault where you can visit it any time you wish without trying to hold it in your memory. When you keep it all in your head, it's stressful. It creates a sense of unease and guilt for all that you aren't getting done. These tasks just pop up in your brain from time to time (all the time) and remind you how ineffective you are, which makes you feel guilty. It's not good, and it's not healthy. Our modern lives are complex enough without the weight of endless tasks that we don't get done.

Step 3:

Once you've got your definitive list, which could amount to 150 to 250 things, take a ten-minute break. No checking emails or anything. Just relax. Then review the list and assign each task a number 1, 2, or 3.

- Ones are big important tasks or projects that, if you could complete them, would give you great gain.

- Twos are important tasks but not as important or urgent as ones.

- Threes are even less important and shouldn't be done before the ones and twos.

Step 4:

Remove the twos and the threes and put them on a separate list that you set aside. Don't get rid of it, just put it to the side. You'll want to keep it accessible for review later, but for now, allow them to exit your mind so you can relax.

Step 5:

You now have the list of your ones, which is still too much to tackle. Repeat the exercise again, ranking the list into ones, twos, and threes. What are the big, important most essential tasks with by far the most gain if you accomplish them? Give them a I. Work hard to whittle down to no more than ten of these. Then, assign a 2 or a 3 to the other tasks.

Step 6:

Remove the twos and threes like you did before, and place that list on top of the original twos and threes list for safe keeping.

Step 7:

Take another short break of about seven minutes.

Step 8:

Review your list of ones and rank them in order of most important to least important, assigning them numbers I through 10.

Step 9:

Focus on numbers I, 2, and 3. Put numbers 4 through 10 on top of the pile with the twos and threes from the previous exercises.

As you plan and execute on these top three priorities, you'll begin to accomplish them. You will, if you stay focused, accomplish more than you ever have before. By the time a year passes, you'll have completed your top ten tasks. And here's the great secret: You'll get 90 percent of the gain you need when you accomplish these ten tasks. The other 140 or 240 won't matter. You won't get them done, and if you review them, you'll find out many are irrelevant and have become obsolete. You just completed your should-do list, and you won't believe how good it feels.

Keep at it. Attack your list, and do it over and over again.

It's deceptively simple because it's just a list that you rank. You'll be tempted to think, "I know this. I know how to do this. What's the big deal?" That's the deceptive part. Odds are you'll be like most people and won't do it. You may plan to get around to it, but here's the thing. If you don't do it, years will go by, one spinning into the next, and you won't have accomplished the most important things.

Your One Thing

A goal that isn't specific, time-bound, charged with emotion, and written down is just wishful thinking.

Remember your *why*? What do you care about? What's the purpose of your practice, your career? What is it that fuels your passion, the thing that you care about the most? It's not money. Money's wonderful. Money makes all things possible. Money equals freedom, but it isn't your *why*.

I want to share a concept I learned from Gary Keller in his book *The One Thing: The Surprisingly Simple Truth Behind Extraordinary Results*. He suggests that we ask this focusing question: What's the one thing I can do such that, by doing it, everything else is easier or unnecessary?

Can we get down to that absolute, most important *one thing*? We have so many goals: personal goals, business goals, financial goals, health goals, and fun goals. In fact, I developed those five categories years ago, and they haven't changed because I can't figure out anything better. This is what our lives contain: personal, business, financial, health, and fun. But, what's *the one thing*?

Keller talks about the one thing, and people get very confused about this because they wonder, "Is there just *one* one thing, or are their *multiple* one things?" I hate to tell you this, but there are multiple one things. And there is also one *truly one thing* that we must find and use as our focus.

This is vital because, when you write down your goals, you'll struggle because you'll think, "I've got these financial goals and these business goals, but I have other goals that are more important to me. They're much nearer and dearer to my heart."

A business goal as your one thing seems crass, and for most of us, it's not the most important thing. Most often, our most important goals are spiritual or family-related. But if you focus on these as your one thing, your business can suffer, and then everything else suffers.

I struggled as I tried to figure out what my one thing is. I asked myself, "What's the one thing that if I could do it right, it would make everything else either unnecessary or much, much easier?" Andrew Carnegie revealed his answer to this question to me as I read his story in Napoleon Hill's masterpiece, *Think and Grow Rich*. Carnegie's top purpose—he called it his definiteness of purpose—his *one thing* as we define it, was to build the greatest steel company in the world, and that's what he did when he built U.S. Steel.

That was his one thing.

Only through that accomplishment could he become one of the great philanthropists of all time. He established libraries all over the United States, universities, and much, much more. What Andrew Carnegie accomplished and the legacy he left is incredible, and it all came to be because he built U.S. Steel. The company he built funded it all.

So, doctor, your one thing has to be **to build the best practice in your region**. In, for instance, the entire southwest, not just your city.

THE PURPOSE OF YOUR PRACTICE IS TO SERVE YOU AND TO FUND YOUR IDEAL LIFESTYLE.

You need to build the best possible practice that you can. You have to be serious. Your practice is your one thing because only it can support and fund everything else in your life that you hold so dear. The purpose of your practice is to serve you and to fund your ideal lifestyle, not the other way around.

You have to be specific about this. How will you measure this? How will you know when you've accomplished what it is that you want? When will that be completed in all areas of your life? You're not just a business; you're a human. You have your personal life, your financial life, your health, your fun—all of it.

My one thing is to build Top Practices into the absolute best company I can conceive of it to be and more. You have to have your one thing, and there can only be one. You can use the focusing question for the one thing and all the other areas of your life and every goal that you write, but you've got to know your one thing. Start with your one thing, and your one thing is your practice. Period. That's what will allow everything else come to fruition.

Writing Goals That Inspire and Motivate

What's the one thing you can do that, by doing it, everything else is easier or unnecessary in the categories of personal, business, financial, health, and fun? How can you accomplish your goals in these areas?

I suggest you use the Top Practices Goal Worksheets, and you can find them on the Top Practices website. They're set up so that you can work backward from your lifetime goal to the current twelve-week period. You should always be able to draw a straight line all the way from your lifetime goal to your three-year vision to your twelve-week plans.

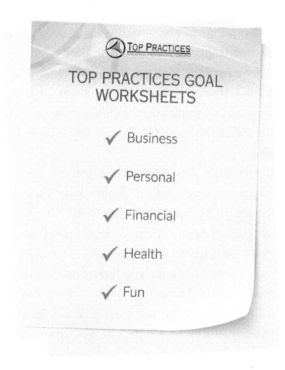

You need to set goals in all the important areas of life because, like everyone, you need balance to be successful. It's imperative that your goals inspire you so much that they'll get you through all the challenges that will come.

And your goals have to be smart. They must be very specific: who, what, when, where, how, and why. For example, a general goal would be to get in shape, but a specific goal would be to join a health club, work out three days a week, and achieve specific measurements in weight and BMI. Goals have to be measurable. Establish the criteria, so you'll know when you hit your numbers. You must hit your benchmarks. They have to be attainable, they have to be realistic, and they have to state when you'll complete them.

Here's a wonderful mind hack that I learned from my friend Dave Frees. Add these two phrases to every goal you create: "or more" and "or sooner." If you have a goal to build your revenues to $2 million in 2020, write "to generate $2 million or more in revenue by December 31, 2020, or sooner."

Now it's time to get busy. Download the goal worksheets and write your goals for your personal life, your business, your career, your financial goals, your health goals, and your fun goals. Move through them by sections. Start with your lifetime goals.

Be sure to think through what you want, not what you think *other people* want or what you think you *should* do. You have to have a burning desire to achieve this. You have to care so much that you'll keep at it no matter what.

Goal work isn't easy. When you try to sort this stuff out, it can be difficult. You might get stuck with thoughts like, "I want world peace," or, "I want to be the richest person in the world." It's hard. We all have an enormous amount of hesitation to do this. Sometimes, the goals you write are just your best guess. It's your dream. I always say that goals are best written in pencil because you'll change them again and again.

I frequently change and adjust my goals. In fact, I've never achieved the goals that I wrote down. I always achieve a different goal, often a better goal, and very often in a different way than I thought I would when I originally created it. As you adapt and reinvent and work on these goals, they'll grow ever clearer. No matter what, persevere. And when they end up in your rearview mirror, you'll think, "Where do I go now?" That's fun!

As you put your dreaming hat on, everything will come into focus. It always does. Sometimes you have goals that are already clear. But, always ask yourself, "Are these goals big enough, are they daring enough, are they fulfilling enough that they will give me joy when I hit them?"

Once you've identified your lifetime goals, look at them and ask, "Where do I need to be in three years if I'm to achieve this by the time I said I would?" All your three-year goals have to be connected to your lifetime goal. If they aren't, something's wrong. If a goal doesn't help you achieve the larger goal, did you miss something?

Don't do the twelve-week goals now; we'll worry about them later. They are execution plans. Right now, focus on your lifetime, three-year, and one-year goals.

Let's address your personal goals first because this is the area where people struggle the most. Personal goals include spiritual goals for yourself, church-related goals, and meditation-related goals. They include relationships with those you love and other people who are important to you. They're about homes that you own or college for your children. These are the kind of goals that don't fall into the other main areas, and they matter. This is your life.

Your business goals are those things that you work on all the time, such as the number of offices, the number of doctors, the amount that you collect, what you take home—all those kinds of things. Believe it or not, this is also the time to set goals for your exit plan. Whether you just started your practice or if you're in the latter part of your career, you need to have an exit plan. If you don't know what that is now, that's okay. Ask yourself, "What would be the coolest thing that could happen?" Write that down. Play with that. Think about that. Ruminate on that.

Now about your fun goals. Everybody wants to skip the fun goals because they think they're not serious and they're not very important.

Wrong!

Nothing could be further from the truth. Without your fun goals, like your vacations or learning to fly an airplane or painting or putting like a golf pro, life can be pretty mundane and routine. We Americans are terrible at taking vacations and protecting our downtime because we think we're so important that our businesses can't run without us.

Trust me, we're not.

You must recharge your batteries. At the end of your life, you won't remember most of the other goals you achieve. The only thing you'll have are the memories of those fun goals, of the things you did with the people you love.

In 2007, when we started Top Practices, Diane wanted to take our girls to Europe. We wanted to go to Paris and London. We started Top Practices in January with nothing. I had savings I could rely on for a time, but we started our business from scratch in January, so how could we take a European vacation in June?

That's not the time to take a vacation. I mentioned this to Diane. I told her I thought we should conserve our funds. And, Diane asked, "What will we remember in ten years? Will we remember that we saved that money and did whatever, or will we remember that we took the girls to Europe?"

And, what do you know, I remember that we took the girls to Europe. In fact, it changed their lives. Annie met her future husband on that fateful trip. Fun stuff.

Plan your next trip. Travel happens to resonate with me because Diane and I like to see the world. We set a goal years ago to visit all the wine-producing regions in the world, and we're well on our way.

I always said we'd start our tour of the world wineries on May 10, 2012, in Bordeaux in front of Chateau Lafite Rothschild in France. I picked that day because it's my birthday. And guess what? I haven't been to Bordeaux yet, but we'll get around to it. However, we've been to over 160 wineries in Napa, we've been to Oregon, to Washington State, to Italy multiple times, along with Portugal, Argentina, Austria, and Champagne. Australia, South Africa, and Spain are also on our list because that's what gives us joy.

If you don't care about travel, then fine; plan something else. Maybe you want an RV that you can take somewhere, or you want to go fishing, or buy a cabin in Utah. Whatever it is, write it down and get started. And for goodness sake, involve the people you love. Don't freak out. Have fun and enjoy this; it's your life.

Next comes your financial goals. What do you want? You should want to be financially independent when you retire. What does that look like to you, and when will that be? Write down your three-year vision. Where do you need to be? You have to start that work now.

In terms of your health goals, what's the point of all this if you don't have your health? Figure out what your lifetime goals are and where you need to be in three years to achieve them.

Sit with this. Work with this. Think about it. Where do you need to be in three years to have the things that you want?

PROSPERITY TIPS:

- If your goals aren't written down, they're mere wishes.

- Focus on your goal and business development work in the summer.

- Use the DSYEP tool to get organized and stay organized.

- The purpose of your practice is to serve you and to fund your ideal lifestyle. Remember that!

DISCUSSION QUESTIONS:

- Are your goals written down, and do you regularly review them? If not, why not?

- How can you change your schedule to give yourself time to work on your goals?

- Why do you go to work each day? What's in it for you?

STEERING YOUR PRACTICE

A bad system will outperform good people with no system 100 percent of the time.

—WARREN BUFFET

My goal wasn't to write a book about management and systems. But there are serious flaws in how we educate professionals in our country. We produce skilled clinicians with extraordinary talents to heal their patients, but we fail to offer them a single course on how to be successful in business. Consequently, most only learn the most basic business practices on the job. They learn from someone who learned how to run a practice from someone else who just tried to do the best with what they had.

It doesn't make sense. It's similar to our K–12 schools, which are charged to prepare our future citizens but don't teach them basic life skills like how to balance a checkbook, how to purchase a home, how money works, how to buy insurance, how to evaluate information and make independent decisions, the tools of entrepreneurship, and on and on. It makes no sense because having these skills is a leading indicator of success.

Doctors graduate, join a practice, and learn how to struggle from a struggling colleague who employs them. This works at first because low volume equals lower complexity, and inefficient systems can get the job done in a reasonable period of time. But as the volume increases, the

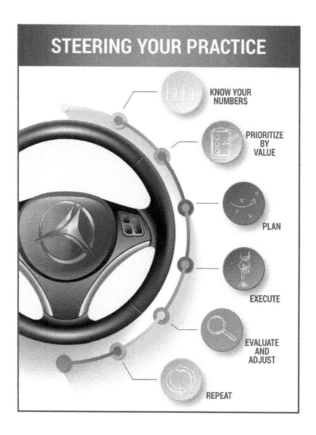

office becomes more and more buried under the management burdens of the business. And to be clear, to operate a medical practice in the U.S. system is complex. In fact, it's ridiculous. Because of the system, medical offices spend an excessive amount of time just trying to get paid.

WITHOUT A MANAGEMENT SYSTEM THAT SUPPORTS AND GUIDES YOUR STAFF, WITHOUT SMART EXPERTS WHO CAN SHOW YOU THE WAY AND TELL YOU WHAT TO DO (AS WELL AS WHAT NOT TO DO), MARKETING AND MINDSET WON'T GET THE JOB DONE FOR YOU.

Michael Gerber, in his classic, *The E-Myth Revisited: Why Most Small Businesses Don't Work and What to Do About It,* discussed the complexity that small businesses face and how the skills of, in our case, the doctors, are not enough to run and manage a profitable, enjoyable medical practice. They need a system that supports and guides their practices.

Without a management system that supports and guides your staff, without smart experts who can show you the way and tell you what to do (as well as what not to do), marketing and mindset won't get the job done for you. That's why I address the essential topic of management now.

Here's a simple way to steer your practice.

Know Your Numbers

Your key performance indicators (KPIs) are metrics and benchmarks to help you discern if your practice is healthy or in a state of dis(ease). Knowing these metrics is essential for anyone who wants to manage their practice and have a personal life.

Here's a short list of your vital KPIs. Your staff needs to report these figures to you weekly, so you can review your progress and take appropriate actions to correct any problems and to enhance the good stuff.

- New Patients Last year
- New Patient Goal for This Year
- New Patients This Year

- Total Patients Last Year
- Total Patient Goal for This Year
- Total Patients This Year

- Total Billed Last Year
- Total Billed Goal for This Year
- Total Billed This Year

- Total Collected Last Year
- Total Collected Goal for This Year
- Total Collected This Year

Track all these goals by month. That means you compare January's numbers *last year* to January's numbers *this year.* You can't compare

January to October. They'll be different, and as you track this year over year, you'll begin to discern the seasonality of your numbers.

In addition to these key numbers, you must calculate your Per Visit Revenue or PVR. This is done by dividing total collections by total number of patient visits for a specific period. You should know your PVR for the previous twelve months and for the previous three months, not month by month. It's just one number for the previous year and one number for the previous three months. You can then compare your last quarter to your yearly number to see if there's a variance.

Knowing your PVR is one of the most powerful points of leverage in your practice. The national average is $95. Most healthy practices range from $120–$220. You will raise your PVR through better management systems and protocols that allow you to practice more comprehensively, raise patient outcomes, and increase your profitability. Raising your PVR even $5 can increase what you pay yourself by thousands of dollars. Managing your practice better makes your patients happier and healthier, and it does the same thing for you.

You can also track your Per Visit Charges (PVC). This is calculated by dividing total billing for a specific period by total patient visits. This is a key number to know because your PVR will be a percentage of what your PVC is. Typically, that is around 55 percent. Most practices collect around 55 percent of what they bill. Your percentage might be different because of how you bill, but if you know your own percentage benchmark, you can monitor it. If there's a sudden change, you can immediately investigate the cause. In the case of precipitous drops, it often involves a problem with a payer or a biller. This percentage indicator is "a canary in the coal mine" because it's an early warning indicator of a problem that will affect your cash flow.

SO OFTEN DOCTORS FIRST DISCOVER THAT SOMETHING'S WRONG WITH THEIR COLLECTIONS WHEN THEY SEE THAT THERE'S NO MONEY IN THE CHECKBOOK. BY THE TIME THIS HAPPENS, THE PROBLEM IS MONTHS OLD, AND REAL HAVOC ENSUES.

So often doctors first discover that something's wrong with their collections when they see that there's no money in the checkbook. By the time this happens, the problem is months old, and real havoc ensues.

This is because it's complicated for doctors to get paid, and it's a basic business principle they never learned from anyone.

Another early warning sign of trouble is your Accounts Receivables (A/R). Every accounting program can produce these reports that show how much money is owed to you. They're organized by time like this:

- 0–30 days
- 30–60 days
- 60–90 days
- 90–120 days
- 120+ days

You should review your A/R at least twice a month. The 0–30 day number should be as big as it can be. This reflects your current business, which you want to be as large as possible. That's why you market your practice.

- 30–60 days should drop off to no more than 25 percent of your total A/R
- 60–90 days should be less than 10 percent
- 90–120 days should approach 0 percent
- 120+ days must be 0 because you are unlikely ever to collect this money owed to you

Smart business owners look at their profit and loss statements and their balance sheet every month. It is not hard to learn to read these reports. Anyone can do it in thirty minutes. Once you understand these essential and foundational business tools, you'll be able to rest easier at night. You'll know you're informed about the health of your company. And you can take actions to make it even healthier.

While there are even more numbers to know, the list isn't endless. Learn how to understand and use these numbers to market and manage your practice more effectively. Do not collect these numbers yourself.

CEOs don't compile reports; they read them and then review them with their teams to take action. Never do this yourself. Have your staff prepare, share, and help interpret these numbers with you.

Prioritize by Value

In the last chapter, we talked about how to get a handle on all the tasks before you by using the Deceptively Simple Yet Extremely Powerful tool for getting organized. This is a key component of steering your practice. Do the important things first and do only the important things.

Plan and Execute

Now, you can get out your goals (lifetime, three-year, and one-year) and begin to break them down into your twelve-week goals.

In his book, *The 12 Week Year: Get More Done in 12 Weeks than Others Do in 12 Months*, Brian Moran suggests that you execute in twelve-week plans, not yearly plans. When the clock's almost out of time, and you can see the scoreboard, you get more done. It's a simple premise: Plan your project tasks for the next twelve weeks, and then accomplish the weekly tasks.

The beauty of this is you know right away if you're serious or not about these plans because you'll track your progress every week. If you don't get things done the first week, you either need to regroup, accomplish it the next week, or accept that fact that you don't care enough about these goals to become happier and wealthier. This is an enormous competitive advantage because 95 percent of people do the bare minimum to get by and then struggle and complain about it to anyone who will listen. Don't let that be you.

It's as simple as that.

Execution is another key to progress. Here are my top execution tools:

1. Twelve-week plans

2. Action plans—these are simple lists that define the task, who's responsible for completing the task, and the date it's to be

accomplished. I've used these for years, and they are my pre-ferred tool to manage both projects and the people responsible for these projects. Here are my rules for action plans:

a) You don't maintain the action plans for the people who do the work. *They* are responsible for managing, updating, and distributing the action plans. When you do this work for them, your people are disempowered. They want and enjoy this level of responsibility. It helps them do good work.

b) No one can remove a task from an action plan without agree-ment by you and any affected team members. You should warn your people that removing tasks from an action plan is a serious offense. I'm a pretty sharp guy, but I can't remember anything on the seven or so action plans that my teams and I work from. If someone removed an item, I wouldn't know, and then at some point I'd have to ask what happened to it. So, I compare last week's action plan to this week's plan to make sure nothing dropped off that I wasn't aware of.

c) No one, including me, can come to a meeting and say, "I didn't get a task done" that was due to be completed. It's another offense that can get you fired because it's that important.

The rule in Top Practices is **No Surprises**. No surprises means that the moment you realize a task won't get done, you inform the team. I tell my people, "You can bring anything to me, and what we will do is either move the deadline further out because it isn't critical or readjust our priorities and assets to get it accomplished. We'll move other dead-lines back for less critical tasks."

This is called *management*. Let's manage the practice together as a team and end the frustration of things never getting done. If you ever catch yourself asking, "What happened with that?" you aren't using action plans because they eliminate that problem. I hate it when my team agrees to a course of action or a plan and someone says, "I'll take care of that." And we all assume he or she will, only to find out they forgot about it almost immediately. Then when we ask about it, he or she says, "Oh I forgot that. I'll do it right away." I hate that. Action plans end that problem forever. In my opinion, they're the single most valuable management tool in the history of human endeavor.

A word about meetings: I used to hate meetings because I thought they got in the way of people doing work until I learned that well-run meetings are *where* the work actually gets done.

You can certainly have too many meetings, but weekly meetings that are organized by an agenda, a time limit, and action plans can be tremendous tools for growth. A well-run meeting has a facilitator who has two primary roles:

- respect and protect the agenda

- stop unnecessary discussions that don't accomplish the agenda

A well-run meeting has an agenda with a start and end time. Some meetings are best held standing up, and much can be accomplished in a ten-minute stand-up meeting. The agenda should be driven by a review of the team's current action plan, task by task. Items are discussed, possibly removed because they are completed, or changed because of the challenges the team faces.

In the beginning, your action plans might be lengthy, and your meetings might run long if the problems are significant. Once, when I assumed responsibility for operations that included a warehouse, I had four-hour meetings with the team every day for about six weeks. Things were that bad. The pushback I got from that plan was huge at first, but we kept at it. We went from there to shorter meetings less frequently until we finally settled into a weekly one-hour meeting. Meetings are where the good work gets done.

Evaluate and Adjust

Everything comes back to your numbers. Once you know your numbers, prioritize your projects, plan, and then execute those plans. Continue to get weekly reports on your key numbers so you can evaluate your progress, identify your challenges, and focus your attention.

The hardest thing to do is to be consistent with this, over and over, forever. Humans get bored, routines can become stale, and we stop useful activities because we lose focus. This happens to us in all facets of our lives, and we must guard against just "phoning it in." Never stop reviewing your

THE HARDEST THING TO DO IS TO BE CONSISTENT WITH THIS OVER AND OVER, FOREVER.

numbers. Find joy in knowing what's going on and continually adjust and grow. Nothing stays the same, and if you're vigilant, you can be prepared for anything life sends your way. As an example, I've shared the DSYEP tool with thousands of people. Many have told me they did it and it found it very helpful. A surprising number then said, "I think I should probably do it again."

Do ya think?

Remember, circumstances always change. A competitor dies, and their office closes. A new group opens up across the street or across town. Review your to-dos and your goals because it's the only way to stay sharp and focused for the rest of your life.

Then repeat.

PROSPERITY TIPS:

- Know your numbers.

- Prioritize by value.

- Plan and execute in twelve-week blocks.

DISCUSSION QUESTIONS:

- How can you gather and review your key numbers weekly? Who will help you?

- Since you can't do everything at once, where will you begin?

- Try to recall a time when you accomplished a task or a project. How did you do it?

ARE WE ALL DOOMED?

Don't worry about the world coming to an end today...
It's already tomorrow in Australia.

—CHARLES M. SCHULTZ

I t would be a gross oversight for a book about business success to overlook the importance of mindset. There are hundreds of books that put their spin on this topic and, even though it seems impossible to add anything new to this discussion, I will try.

There's a reason that everyone who writes or teaches people success strategies talks about mindset, both the positive and negative aspects of it. It's because your mindset is the most important factor for achieving both personal and professional success. In his classic book, *Think and Grow Rich*, Napoleon Hill stressed the vital importance of a Positive Mental Attitude (PMA). He made it one of his foundational principles. Hill observed that everything works better and produces greater results when combined with a Positive Mental Attitude. Everything!

I've certainly observed this in my own life and career. People see their lives and circumstances through either a positive or negative filter. Very few people have a neutral filter, and from what I've seen, that would be dangerous because it would mean they didn't care.

In my work with doctors and their staff in Top Practices, I mainly see positive mindsets. Ninety percent of my members have positive mindsets. There's a reason for that. Negative people aren't drawn to the message and methods of Top Practices. It's like a bright light that hurts their eyes, and they turn away. I'm always surprised by the number of people who see things so negatively. Most of them don't realize they're like this, and they'd tell you they're a positive person. But what determines a positive or negative attitude is how they perceive their circumstances and describe them to others.

It's always someone else's fault. The government, insurance companies, their partners, their staff, their patients, their communities, their spouses—always someone else.

Few people have a positive mindset, but when you find them, it inspires you, and it's infectious. The most successful members of Top Practices have positive mindsets, or at least they aspire to that. One of my best moments was when one of my doctors introduced me to his colleague. He said, "This is Rem Jackson, the CEO of Top Practices. When I met him, I was a negative person, and now I'm a positive person." I beamed with pride when he said that. If I can impact anyone in that way, then my work is worth it. And it *is* worth it. It's been staggering to see the number of people who've changed their lives by transforming their mindsets, then their actions, and then their results.

We all have the seeds of any greatness we desire inside us. Most of us have been battered so many times by negative messages from the media, from friends, family, and others who're supposed to love and support us. But they don't have it in them to love and support us, so we've lost the belief that we can accomplish whatever we want.

WE ALL HAVE THE SEEDS OF ANY GREATNESS WE DESIRE INSIDE US.

Napoleon Hill's great secret, his key to everything, was, "Whatever the mind can conceive and believe, it can achieve." It's that simple, and it's that powerful. I've known since childhood that I'd be a happy, successful person. When I faced setbacks and challenges—some significant, as we all have—I just *knew* I'd be successful. And so, it came to pass because nothing else was an option. Other people I've known have always given in to fear and worry and believed that they wouldn't succeed. That, too, came to pass.

You control your own thoughts. You are in charge, and no one can get in your head unless you let them.

Recognize, as wise people do, that you are not your body. Your body is a wonderful tool, but when it passes, you persist.

Recognize that you are not your mind. This one is harder. Your mind is a tool just like your body, and its job is to keep you safe and solve problems. When you identify with a busy, worried, fearful mind, you become disturbed and anxious. One of the best books you can read that discusses this in detail is *The Power of Now: A Guide to Spiritual Enlightenment* by Eckhart Tolle.

Learn that you are the observer of the mind, and you can quiet your mind when you notice it running amuck. Just smile and thank it for its good work, and then think about nothing for a mere second or two (or longer). Give it a rest and focus on now, not the past or future, just now. When you short circuit all the rumination, you can go deeper into relaxed focus and get some stuff done. Try it. And when you do, always do it from a positive mindset. It's always better and much more productive and powerful.

Your subconscious mind is your number one asset and ally. Your conscious mind is but a small percentage of your total mind. Your subconscious mind is an incredible supercomputer that has only one function: to help you. Your subconscious mind never argues with you. It exists solely to help your conscious mind accomplish whatever it tells it to do, which is why it's so important to be careful about what you think. Your subconscious is always listening and will support whatever you're thinking. If you're worrying or are fearful and expecting the worst, your subconscious mind will do its best to bring that to fruition. Your minute-to-minute thoughts are vitally important. Don't focus on your worries and fears; instead, think about the blessings and positives you are working to achieve.

Napoleon Hill talked to his subconscious mind. He called him "sub." He would give him tasks and assignments. He would say, "Sub, I've got a job for you. I want you to figure this out for me." He claims the title *Think and Grow Rich* came to him at 3:00 a.m. after he tasked "sub" to come up with a million-dollar title for his book.

I've adopted this same practice. I speak to my "sub" multiple times a day. I encourage him to keep me focused on positive things and ask him to remove my worries and negative thoughts and replace them with the good I'm working toward. Before I go to bed, I remind him to prevent me from ruminating on things that disturb me and, instead, to find solutions. It works. It's remarkable. I couldn't live without my relationship with this incredible ally, friend, supporter, and supercomputer. Just try this yourself. You'll see results almost immediately, and you'll never want to stop. I promise.

Are we all doomed? If you watch the twenty-four-hour news and opinion cycles, you'll think we are. The media loves to work us up. It sells more commercials for them. The real problem is that when you obsessively watch your favorite opinion news show or listen to talk radio, you outsource your thoughts to someone else—and they have an agenda. Ask yourself, "Why do they take the positions they take and is any of it based in fact?"

Facts matter. The truth matters. The opinion news entertainers are engaged in something, but it isn't informing us. The more outrageous they are, the more money they make.

Unplug from all of it. Start with unplugging from most of it and then move to a complete blackout of entertainment news. You'll feel much more peaceful and cleansed. You'll find hours returned to you and your friends and family. People will mention the most recent news crisis, and you won't even know about it. Better yet, you won't care. You can spend your time growing rich. Rich in relationships and love. Rich in enjoying your days. Rich in building a business that provides for and supports your emotional and financial health first so you can care for the emotional and financial health of your loved ones.

You can extend that circle even further to your patients and any other people you meet. You might even try to write a book to extend your positive influence beyond your current reach. You might even call it *Podiatry Prosperity*.

In spite of everything you read and hear, we aren't all doomed. Had I been alive and aware in the late 1930s and 1940s, I would have thought the world couldn't recover from the horror of World War Two. And yet it did. And it does. And it will.

Here's an idea: When you wake up every morning, smile as soon as you open your eyes. This small smile, which is my first conscious act every morning, is a trigger to remind me to focus on the blessings of my life and to live each moment in the present. I don't worry about or regret the past. I no longer fret about the future, which never arrives because we're always in the present moment.

Banish fear from your life. I've heard fear defined as False Events Appearing Real, and that is a perfect definition.

The United States has been a hot, crazy mess since 1776. It will be just the same in 2076. And I wouldn't want to start a business anywhere else. Even with all the ridiculous interference in medical practices that seems to get worse every day, our system is designed to more than reward you for your positive mindset and proactive work to serve your patients. The more you stay focused on service to your patients, your staff, your community, and above all, your family, the happier you will be.

THE TIGER AND THE SPIDER

On a beautiful summer morning, a tiger took a walk in his jungle. He stumbled upon a gazelle nibbling on a leaf in a clearing with the sunlight streaming everywhere. The sight of the gazelle reminded him that he hadn't eaten in a long time. The gazelle suddenly looked like lunch!

Quietly stalking the animal, the tiger finally pounced and easily brought down the feast he enjoyed for the rest of the afternoon. Finally, completely full, he decided it was time for a nice long tiger nap. He spied the opening to a cave and hopped in. The cave was dry and very comfortable. He jumped into another opening and found the perfect space for a tiger to take a nap. He turned in a circle several times and laid down in the perfect spot and quickly went to sleep.

He slept for a very long time. While he was sleeping, a little spider wandered into the same small cave and saw the opening in the very alcove in which the tiger was sleeping.

"What a perfect place to spin a web!" she thought.

She carefully spun a gorgeous web that covered the entire opening and waited for her prey.

Many hours later, long after the little spider had had her fill and left, the tiger woke up. He felt refreshed and ready for another day in his jungle. He gazed at the opening, now covered with the spider's web, and sat back on his haunches.

"Where is the opening?" he wondered. "It was right there when I jumped in, but now it's gone!" He became alarmed and started pacing and searching for the opening. "It has to be here somewhere!"

He searched and searched for days and became increasingly frightened and weak. After a very long time, he laid in the same spot where he took his nap and became a pile of bones. No longer the king of his jungle, he had been brought down by his thoughts alone. At any time, he could have easily hopped through the wisp of a web built by the spider, walked out the door, and found his next meal. Instead, he saw a barrier in front of him he believed he couldn't go through, and he died.

Is it time to change the way you see your situation and simply walk through the web with all your strength, tenacity, courage, and power to accomplish your dreams and goals?

PROSPERITY TIPS:
- Everything in your life is determined by your mindset.

- You can achieve anything you desire. You've always had that ability.

- Unplug from the twenty-four-hour entertainment news, and instead, feed your mind with positive ideas.

- Stop worrying. You've always landed on your feet and you always will.

DISCUSSION QUESTIONS:
- Do you consider yourself a strong person with a positive mindset—yes or no? Regardless of your answer, why did you answer the way you did?

- List three things you've achieved in your life that weren't easy.

- How much time do you spend every day focused on entertainment news? Is it helping you to be more informed? Is it making you happier?

- How much time do you spend reviewing the past or worrying about the future?

WHAT YOUR INNER SIX-YEAR-OLD CAN TEACH YOU ABOUT SUCCESS

Be your own best friend each and every day.

—REM JACKSON

Our lives can be complex, frustrating, and difficult. Or simple and blessed. Sometimes it seems like they're both at the same time. So much depends on your inner life and mindset. You must remember that there's no point in rehashing the past because it no longer exists, and there's no point in worrying about the future because it never comes. You can only live in the present moment, and when you do that, you have a decent chance for a life filled with grace, peace, and happiness.

I want to share a simple exercise with you that's helped me as much as anything I've ever learned.

Your Inner Six-Year-Old

Who talks trash to you? I mean the really nasty stuff—the words that give you a psychological blow to the gut? Most likely, it's not the people you work with. They're far too skilled to beat you up openly. Not your family (hopefully), at least not directly. Those messages, if they do come, can produce guilt, but they aren't the really horrible stuff.

Nope. We're the only ones who can take ourselves out to the wood-shed and open up a big can of whoop-ass. No one can grind our souls into dust like we can do to ourselves. We're all guilty of this, and some of us are fantastically gifted in this category.

I'd like to ask you why. Why do you do that to yourself? What did you do that was so bad that you deserve to be psychologically beaten?

WHY DO YOU DO THAT TO YOURSELF? WHAT DID YOU DO THAT WAS SO BAD THAT YOU DESERVE TO BE PSYCHOLOGICALLY BEATEN?

And make no mistake, that's what is this is, a steady drumbeat of abuse from the one person you can't get away from no matter how you try: yourself.

I know this because I have more than my own share of self-inflicted scars, and I've been like this most of my life. I'm a first born (strike one). I'm an over-achiever type (strike two). And I care what people think about me (strike three).

I've got my reasons to be so hard on myself, and so do you. One of those reasons is that I was a bit of a disappointment to my father because I was a terrible athlete. I'm not like my father, who was a talented high-school heavyweight wrestler and a defensive tackle on the football team. He even had a nickname: the Philipsburg Panther. All this is a bit remarkable because he also had polio as a child and has a size seven left foot and a size eleven right foot.

I had a nickname too: worst athlete to ever attend Philipsburg-Osceola High School. (Not true, but it felt that way.)

I had the lead in some of our high school plays (after I quit football), played the piano for the school chorus one year, and had a fun high school rock band named "Sweet Earth" with some friends and my brother Barry on drums. This was all due to my mother, a wonderful music educator and inspiration, not just to my brother and me, but to thousands of people who either studied music with her in elementary school or sang in her choirs.

I had these three strikes against me, as we all do, but I overcame all of them. I became aware of this self-abuse a long time ago, and I now refuse to mistreat myself. I even refuse to let others do it to me.

I'm too busy thinking and growing rich in all parts of my life to allow any room in my mind or spirit for this kind of painful activity. I've spent as much time as I can bombarding my brain with positive books, CDs, masterminds, friends, and music. I stop and smell as many roses as I can, but the most effective technique I've ever used to help me overcome my own verbal bashing was something I discovered myself.

Here it is:

This weekend, wouldn't it be fun if you could spend the day with yourself as a six-year-old? You could drive up to your old house, and there you'd be, on the porch, ready for you to pull up in the car. You'd run up and jump into the car, buckle your seatbelt, and look over at the grown-up ready to hang out with you with great anticipation. Your adult self would look into the eyes of this precious child and ask, "Well, Remy, what would you like to do today?" Of course, you'd already know the secrets of this little child's heart, and when your six-year-old self answered, you'd reply, "I thought you might say that. Let's go!"

As you spent the day with this lovely child, how would you talk to him? You might, of course, try to teach him all about investments and suggest some great stock tips; you might even try to teach him how to access the funds to accomplish the trades. But this six-year-old would be lost, so you'd soon abandon that plan. You might tell him not to go out with a specific girl on a certain night so he could avoid two years of heartache in the future, but this plan would most likely fail as well.

What you wouldn't do is berate and belittle this child. You wouldn't hit him on the forehead and call him stupid. You wouldn't tell him that he "always does this!" You wouldn't wake him up in the middle of the night and pound him with a blow-by-blow parade of his mistakes. You wouldn't repeat the litany of things you were told were wrong with you throughout your life by your family and friends. You wouldn't look at him in disgust for being too short, tall, fat, skinny, average, etc. You wouldn't attack him incessantly with his list of shortcomings.

Instead, you would nurture and cherish that little soul. You would tell him how great he is and how much you love him. You'd tell him about some of the wonderful blessings that will come his way. If you could, you'd tell him about his children and how wonderful they'll be, how he'll become a doctor, and how proud he'll be of that achievement. If you could, you'd tell him that he will help so many people in their careers. You'd tell him about the letters from patients who will tell about the difference he's made in their lives. You would tell him about the blessings that will rain down upon him.

You will tell him that you love him and that he will make mistakes in his life, many, but that he shouldn't be hard on himself when it happens. You will tell him that every time he makes a mistake, he meant to do the right thing. He tried to be the best person he could. And you will tell him that he's a wonderful person worthy of love and respect.

And you'll tell him that **you will always be with him—every minute of every day—and you'll help and guide him. You will always be there for him, and you will never let him down.** And you'll tell him that you love him. Many times.

This little six-year-old will look deep in your eyes and believe every word you say, just like your adult self believes every word you say today.

So, the next time you take yourself out to the woodshed, stop. Remember to speak to yourself as though you are that six-year-old. Resolve never again to inflict pain and suffering on yourself. Shrink yourself down to a little six-year-old and look into those eyes before you speak to yourself. You'll find yourself saying, "It's okay. You weren't trying to mess that up. Let's fix it. It's not that bad. You are a wonderful person, worthy of love and respect."

Keep your promise to that little six-year-old you. Be your own best friend each and every day. Nurture your own spirit and mind and body. Turn to yourself as your number one source of support.

> BE YOUR OWN BEST FRIEND EACH AND EVERY DAY. NURTURE YOUR OWN SPIRIT AND MIND AND BODY. TURN TO YOURSELF AS YOUR NUMBER ONE SOURCE OF SUPPORT.

Celebrate the blessings you have. They are great and many. Stop and smell the roses every time you walk past them.

If you nurture your own spirit, you'll have an almost limitless capacity to help and love others. I've made this one of my top goals.

Diane gave me a wonderful gift for our twentieth wedding anniversary on which she had written some nice words about me. She said, "Remy, you care about us more than it seems humanly possible." I liked that. The only way I could hear that from someone I love is to care about me first. So, I'm here to tell you—this does work.

Nurture your inner six-year-old, and your adult self will be much better for it.

PROSPERITY TIPS:

- Be very kind to yourself. You deserve it.

- Speak to yourself as though you are only six years old and change the conversation to something positive and constructive.

- Be your own best support and cheerleader.

DISCUSSION QUESTIONS:

- How did the story make you feel about your relationship with yourself?

- How can you embrace this kind of generous self-talk? What triggers can you use to remember to do this in moments when you feel low?

STOP WORRYING, DON'T QUIT, AND YOU'LL WIN AT EVERYTHING

The journey of a thousand miles begins with one step.

—LAO TZU

ife isn't easy. We all face struggles and setbacks. I call these setbacks *stink bombs*. When stink bombs go off in your life and business, they don't cause damage, but they smell terrible and cause stress until they begin to dissipate.

Most of us get about three stink bombs per year. Stink bombs aren't the daily problems and challenges we must deal with just because we are alive. Stink bombs are things like the letter from the IRS that says you're being audited. We get upset when these occur, but within two weeks or so, it always gets sorted out.

I talk to too many doctors each month to have any other opinion. It's just how life works. What matters is how you respond. Here's a story that I hope inspires you.

My daughter, Iris, set a goal to be an entertainment lawyer in Los Angeles, and she attended Pepperdine School of Law in Malibu, California. Finding an internship is an essential component in the law school experience, and you might guess that internships are competitive.

At least they are in Los Angeles in the entertainment industry. And Iris wanted to work in entertainment law.

She worked to find an internship and had been rejected everywhere, many, many times. It hadn't worked out for her the previous summer, nor did it work out in the fall or spring semesters. No job, just rejection.

Throughout this time, her mother and I coached and supported her. I gave her a copy of Jeff Olson's book, *The Slight Edge: Turning Simple Disciplines into Massive Success and Happiness*, an outstanding book I give every Top Practices member when they join. I told her to move forward with faith because something would break for her if she simply didn't stop. I also told her that it would most likely happen in a way she didn't expect.

Years earlier, when she was preparing to go to law school, I told her that she only had two jobs: (1) to learn as much as she could and (2) to meet everybody, go to everything, and build her list because that list was the most valuable thing she'd ever possess other than her law license.

She took all that to heart. In her first year, she wanted to attend a seminar at University of Southern California about entertainment law, and we encouraged her to go. She later reported that the content wasn't that useful to her at that point in her education, but she stayed until the end. When she left the seminar, she couldn't find her car in the parking lot. She got lost, as did another woman who'd attended the seminar. This woman was a lawyer for a major movie studio, NBCUniversal. They searched for their cars together, and twenty minutes later, they both found their cars and Iris had the woman's card.

And here's where it gets good. Iris didn't lose the card. She didn't save it to try to connect with the woman later. Iris immediately emailed her, told her she enjoyed meeting her, and said she'd love to take her out for coffee to talk about the law and her career at the studio. The woman not only agreed, but she invited Iris to the historic movie lot where they spent a few hours together.

Time went on, and Iris wished her happy holidays around the end of the year.

In the meantime, Iris ran for vice president of the Women's Legal Association (WLA) at Pepperdine and won. Once elected, she learned that the current president would be leaving at the end of the semester, so Iris would then be the president. Cool. Oh, and all the while she continued to drive all over town for interviews only to hear that someone else had gotten each internship. Very discouraging.

As president of the WLA, she co-organized a mixer between law students and lawyers in the field of entertainment law. A lot of people came. Iris invited every single person who hadn't hired her, intending to ask them if they had any advice about how she might have done better and been selected. The woman who'd been lost with her in the parking lot couldn't make the event, but she asked if Iris was looking for an internship that summer. "Well, yes I am," Iris replied.

"Send me your info, and I'll arrange an interview," came the reply.

Iris booked the appointment and learned that she'd be interviewing on the Universal Lot with thirteen lawyers at one time. She started her internship that summer with NBCUniversal.

It's All About The Slight Edge

Iris could have stayed home that day two years earlier. She could have left the conference early. She could have ignored the woman in the parking lot who was lost like she was. She could have neglected to ask for her card, not followed up, not stay connected to her list—and she could still be looking for that elusive internship.

Later, she found out that over one thousand candidates had applied for that position.

Slight Edge. Faith. Do the small things. Understand the value of the list and connect to it. Funny that life works this way. Life always works this way. Always. Think of all the great things in your life. Almost every single one of them involved some version of you getting "lost in a parking lot," but still following through. Imagine how many of these opportunities we miss because we don't do the small things that will make us successful every day. Just imagine.

People say there are no jobs for graduating lawyers. Well, there are no internships either.

But there are parking lots for you to get lost in—everywhere.

Iris now practices entertainment law in Los Angeles. It works. It just does.

PROSPERITY TIPS:

- We all get at least three stink bombs a year. Expect them.

- There's no such thing as luck, just opportunity meeting preparation.

- Get lost in a parking lot!

DISCUSSION QUESTIONS:

- How have you prepared for the challenges that will inevitably come your way? Will you deal with them or try to avoid them?

- Do you follow up on your plans or do you quit in the middle of something when it gets hard? Why?

- Try to recall a time when you "got lost in a parking lot." What happened?

HOW YOU'LL KNOW WHEN YOU'VE "ARRIVED"

Rivers know this: there is no hurry. We shall get there some day.

—WINNIE-THE-POOH

How will you know when you've arrived? You don't. That's because we don't ever "arrive." That might sound obvious, but I can tell you it's something that most people don't understand.

Most people think that they will be happy "when." We all engage in this kind of thinking, and here are some common ones for doctors:

- I'll be happy when I get into the right college.
- I'll be happy when I get into the right podiatry school.
- I'll be happy when I get the perfect residency.
- I'll be happy when I'm practicing.
- I'll be happy when I own my own practice.
- I'll be happy when I have my practice running well and profitable.
- I'll be happy when I have x number of millions saved up, and I can retire.

The problem is that "when" never comes. There's always another level of success or security to strive for.

In my younger days, I visited people who had beautiful homes and thought how nice it would be to own a home like theirs. Later in my career, I visited homes that had a house just like the house I thought would be my dream house, but it was merely a guest home on their property.

It doesn't matter who you are or what you have, you never arrive. There's always a nicer house, a better situation, or something else you need to achieve. Or, if you've achieved what you desire, then the worry and fear of losing it take over, and the same thoughts plague you but now in reverse.

Does money make you happy? The answer is "yes" and "no."

It's "yes" if you're so poor you don't have food, safety, or shelter. If you can make enough money to obtain these three things, you become much happier. After that and all the way to the level of people like Jeff Bezos, there's no difference in happiness. Money doesn't make you happier after your basic needs are met.

In fact, to win the lottery can often be a curse. People who win the lottery are often back to their original financial position within seven years. They just can't believe there's a world in which they are financially independent, so they behave in ways that sabotage their windfall and restore them to their true self-image.

I enjoy coaching my doctors when they worry about "the bubble is going to burst" syndrome. This happens when they achieve a level of financial success, and they've sorted out their business systems so that their practice is on time, profitable, and efficient. They then begin to worry that something's wrong, that there's a bubble that will burst, and that their troubles will start again. The fact is, there isn't a bubble; they've just forgotten how to be at peace. They've become so accustomed to stress and guilt that it's become the normal state for them. They've forgotten what it's like to live well and be in the present moment.

Happiness and the reduced stress level that accompanies it can be very disconcerting for those of us who've struggled with high levels of stress. Life with some stress is normal, so I like to use this water test to help judge the stress level. How high is the water you're standing in?

- Is it up to your neck?
- Is it chest-high?
- Is it waist-high?

- Is it at your knees?
- Is it up to your ankles?

This is a good way to gauge how you feel. The water level always moves. Things happen.

So how do I deal with all these issues—daily problems, annoyances, frustrations, and stink bombs? It's through my commitment to live in what I call a state of "Peace of Mind." Here's how I do that. I know that in twenty-four hours, whatever made me upset will be resolved, and I'll be back to that peace of mind I strive for, so I decide not to allow the issue to upset my peace of mind. I grab onto the peace I know I'll have in twenty-four hours anyway. I get to be happy today, right now. And when I claim that peace, I solve the issue better because I'm centered and peaceful. When the stink bombs come, I do the same thing. This takes more effort, but I know I'll be fine in two weeks, so I just remember the peace of mind I'll regain in two weeks and choose to live in it now, in the present moment.

> Happiness is a choice.
> Patience is a choice
> Anger is a choice.
> Love is a choice.

Happiness is a choice. I choose to live in the good old days now. I love being married to Diane, and I choose to live in happily ever after with her now in our house in the desert—not at some point later on when my ship comes in.

Anger is a choice. Thomas Jefferson said, "When angry, count to ten before you speak. If very angry, count to one hundred." Whoever loses their temper in an argument, loses the argument.

Patience is a choice. When you choose patience and try to understand the other person, you'll achieve so much more in the moment. You may find solutions that aren't available to the angry mind. You will take care of yourself.

And in The End...

I wrote this book for podiatrists who want to know how to market and manage their practices. I wrote this book for you if you want to earn the income you deserve and maintain a positive mindset that will change your life. I wrote this book to give you back your nights and weekends. I wrote this book for your family and friends and anyone you love and cherish. When you're at your best, you can help them be their best, too.

I wrote this book for the good people who work in your employ, who stand shoulder-to-shoulder with you every day. They have their own goals and dreams, and as you achieve yours, you will wisely help them achieve theirs. There's no other way.

I wrote this book for your patients. Only by putting yourself first and being your practice's first and healthiest patient can you more profoundly serve others and give them the best possible care.

Podiatry Prosperity is my earnest attempt to share my mission for my Top Practices members with you. We mastermind together every month to raise the bar ever higher in pursuit of our goals and dreams. I invite you to join us.

Love is a choice. In the end, for me, love is the only choice. My best wishes to you on your journey.

PROSPERITY TIPS:

- We never arrive. Life is a journey until we take our final breath.

- Money doesn't make you happy, but being happy can make you a lot of money.

- Choose to be happy, and you will be.

DISCUSSION QUESTIONS:

- How might you be living in the future, waiting for your ship to come in? How can you decide to live in the present instead?

- What's your current level of stress, and how can you begin to manage it?

- How can you turn happiness, anger, patience, and love into choices? How would that change your life and relationships?

WITH THANKS AND GRATITUDE

Gratitude is the fairest blossom which springs from the soul.

—HENRY WARD BEECHER

*P*odiatry Prosperity is the culmination of more than twelve years of working closely with podiatrists, their staff, and dozens of experts in business and marketing. I have many people to thank for their encouragement, support, intelligence, creativity, and friendship.

I must first thank my partner in life and business, Diane Whitman Jackson. Without her belief in me and her talented business mind, I would not have had the skills or courage to launch or run Top Practices. Thank you, Diane, I love you.

I must also thank my three daughters, Emily, Annie, and Iris. My dears, you inspire me every day. You motivate me to be the best man I can be. I love you more than I can ever express.

Before Top Practices launched, the friendship and belief in me that my friend Greg Gilson exhibited put into motion the series of events that would reveal my life's work to me. I will be forever grateful to him. Thank you so much, Greg.

Top Practices would not have launched without Diane's support, but two others were there when everything was only an idea. The first is my friend from childhood, Patrick Chieppor. Pat was in the midst of big career events in his life (all very positive) as I was launching Top

Practices. His business acumen and his support in the early years when I needed it the most were vital to keeping me moving forward. His advice and mentorship every day since then continues to be one of my most treasured resources. Thank you, PJ. I will never forget it.

The second man is one of the few people in my life that I call mentor. Ed Staub taught me much of what I know about business, sales, marketing, and integrity. The phrase "Nurture, Nurture, Nurture" is not original to me. I learned that from Ed. He met with me on January 3, 2007, at a Bob Evans Restaurant in Lancaster, Pennsylvania, and as I told him about Top Practices, he "read my mind" and helped me with every challenge I was facing. Thank you forever, Ed. Thank You.

Greg Gilson introduced me to Hal Ornstein, DPM and the board of trustees of the American Academy of Podiatric Practice Management (AAPPM). Hal immediately saw how I could help the members of the AAPPM. He was my guide, shepherd, and cheerleader for many years. Without Hal, I would never have been able to affect the lives of so many doctors. I've told Hal that he has been an angel in my life as he has been to so many others. Hal, thank you so much. I am forever grateful to you.

There were other doctors at that initial meeting with the AAPPM: Jeff Frederick, DPM; Charlie Greiner, DPM; Bill McCann, DPM who continue to support my mission of lifting up podiatrists and I thank you all. Your commitment to your profession and the support of your fellow doctors inspires me every day.

Dr. John Guliana was not at that first meeting, but I soon met him in Florida at an AAPPM meeting. It was obvious to me at the outset that John was someone special. He is one of the most professional, smart, gracious, talented, high-integrity people I've ever known. John, you have influenced my career and my life more than you realize. Thank you from the bottom of my heart.

You need friends to be successful. You need a mastermind alliance to stay focused and succeed. I met my mastermind alliance about eighteen months before I launched Top Practices. Greg Gilson introduced me to Ben Glass, and Ben told me I had to meet Tom Foster. Ben Glass is a lawyer from Fairfax, Virginia who loves marketing. Ben shared all that enthusiasm with me and endless information. It was through Ben that I found the keys to transforming my God-given talents into a system and a business model that would transform the lives of several thousand people directly and far more indirectly. Thank you, Ben. I remain forever grateful to you for all the friendship, support, and brotherhood you showed me as we both started our companies.

Tom Foster is the CEO of Foster Web Marketing. He knows more about the internet than anyone I know. He is my friend. In the early years, Tom made it possible for Top Practices to flourish with his knowledge, skill, and websites. I am deeply grateful for all of that. But Tom is much more to me than all that. He never wavers in his love for his friends and is simply the definition of a brother. Tom, I love you. Thank you. Thank you.

Speaking of brothers. I have one sibling, my brother, Barry. I've loved Barry longer than anyone except my parents. Barry, my world is so much brighter and fun because you are in it. You are the best brother anyone could ever have. Thank you for just being my brother. I love you.

Life brings people to you in the most interesting ways. In 2010, I met Lori Hibma. Initially working for a podiatrist herself as an office administrator, Lori joined Top Practices as a member. She was active and engaged and involved, and as I got to know her more, she demonstrated how talented she was and how much integrity she possessed. Time moved on, and we began to work together. We wanted to do some of the marketing work for our doctors, and Lori began helping them "just get it done." Over time that necessity has grown into the Virtual Marketing Directors team, which now helps our Top Practices members have the best digital marketing in podiatry. Thank you, Lori, for your skills, and thank you for all that you and your team do every day to support our members. It's been a true blessing.

I realized early on that if I filled Top Practices members' reception rooms with the patients they want and need to see, that it put stress on their management systems. Doctors are not taught business skills, and this is their number one limiter to success. I was teaching them marketing and mindset, but they needed more specific podiatric business skills to turn those patients into profits. Enter Peter Wishnie, DPM; and Tina Del Buono, PMAC.

I first met Peter in 2006, before I launched Top Practices at an AAPPM event I had coordinated. I led a workshop in Columbus, Ohio on practice marketing and growth. About forty people attended that first meeting. At one point, I asked the group if they'd ever written down their goals. Three people raised their hands and said that they had. One of them, Dr. Peter Wishnie of Piscataway, New Jersey, said that he had them with him. Then he reached into his breast pocket and produced them in a nice holder. I could tell that Peter had his act together. But what impressed me the most then and to this day is that he didn't need to show off; he just wanted to learn.

He approached me after the workshop, and we sat down. He explained that he wanted to help other doctors enjoy their careers and make more money, and he wanted to teach as I had all day. We decided to get to know each other to see where things would take us. I didn't know this guy, and even though he passed the smell test, I needed to know much more about him before I would work with him.

Peter joined Top Practices in 2007, as one of the first members. I got to know him and learned how well he runs his practice. It's impressive and it's all about systems. Peter is an avid student of other smart people, and he took good ideas and made them his own. Along the way, he invented quite a few of his own.

We began to offer professional development courses for doctors and their staff in 2010, with Peter leading those courses that focused entirely on his systems and protocols. That grew fast, and we knew we needed to create a way for 24/7 learning for our offices. But we needed one key ingredient: a coach and mentor for our office staff members. While there are very good people out in the marketplace who provide coaching and training about management, there aren't very many, and I needed someone with the same rapport I had with Dr. Wishnie.

That's when I met Tina del Buono. She managed her husband's practice in Santa Rosa, California and consulted with others to help with their practice management. She had the same passion for teaching others that Peter had, and when I kept bumping into her at conferences and hearing her speak, I realized I'd found my mentor for the office staff. She made my day when she said she wanted to work with us, so we launched the Top Practices Virtual Practice Management Institute—a 24/7 resource for medical practice management that includes instruction, coaching, and mentorship from Peter and Tina.

Peter and Tina, thank you for your friendship. Thank you even more for your incredible expertise and passion for teaching others how they can manage their practices and still have a life. I am grateful every day that we work together so closely.

Operating a business can be very enjoyable. One of the gifts it can bring is introductions to people who share your passions but have very different skill sets that extend your own. Two people of special note are Dave Frees and Jay Henderson. Dave is a probate, trusts, and estates attorney in southeastern Pennsylvania. Dave shares the Top Practices Mindset Coaching Call with me every month and is an utter joy to work with. His creativity and expertise, combined with his incredible sense of humor and a servant's heart, have made working together one of the real joys I've had at Top Practices. Thank you, Dave.

Jay Henderson, whose company www.RealTalentHiring.com is an essential resource to our Top Practices members, is another gift of entrepreneurship to me. Jay is a consummate professional who began his career by working with Dr. Stephen Covey. His ability to help us make the right hiring decisions, along with his business experience, is an invaluable resource for our members. Jay once said to me, "Always take the high road." This is one of the single most valuable pieces of advice I've ever received. Taking the high road isn't easy emotionally, but it's always the right thing to do and always produces the best possible outcome. Thank you, Jay, for your friendship and leadership.

In life, certain people seem to be on the journey with you for the entire trip. For me, Dave Ryan is one of those people. I met Dave over thirty years ago at a Christmas dinner for a company for which he, Diane, and I all worked. A friendship ensued, and throughout my career, I've reached out to Dave every time I needed someone 100 percent reliable on the team. Top Practices members know Dave well because his job is to help them in any way he possibly can. He's a role model for so many people who know him and for me. In his role as a lay leader in his church, he's respected for his integrity and message. Dave, thank you for always having my back and for putting our Top Practices members first in all you do.

I must especially thank the doctors of The Top Practices Mastermind Group and the Virtual Practice Management Institute for your earnest support of me and Top Practices' mission. The doctors of Top Practices have shared their entire marketing and management playbook with each other—with no reservations—for the past twelve years. Without your willingness to share the best that you know, it would be impossible for me to deliver on the Top Practices mission. There are just too many of you to name individually. Thank you for allowing me to conduct my life's work. I am deeply grateful for the blessing of serving you every single day.

I want to thank my parents, Rem Jackson, Jr. and Patricia Coldiron. I've looked up to my dad my entire life and always wanted to be just like him. That didn't quite work out because my dad and I are very different people. My desire to live up to his expectations of me has been a driving force that pushed me to the levels of success I've attained. Dad and I became great friends when I became an adult. That love and friendship have only deepened. I love you, Dad. Thank you for all you taught me. Your generosity has inspired me my entire life.

Mom, how do I thank the best mother anyone could ever have? All that is good in me flows directly from my mother. She is a legend in our small town of Philipsburg, Pennsylvania for her music education. Her legacy of music will live forever in central Pennsylvania. Thank you, Mom. You are my biggest fan. My staunchest supporter. You laugh longer and louder at my jokes than anyone. I love you. Without you, none of this would have been possible. Thank you.

One final thank you. Two years ago, Diane met Nancy Erickson, founder of The Book Professor®. Nancy's mission is to help busy people actually write the book they've always wanted to write. When Diane found out what Nancy did, she said, "Rem, you need to talk to Nancy." I did, and through her brilliant approach, *Podiatry Prosperity* was written. Nancy, thank you for your guidance and support. I couldn't have done it without you.

When you work with Nancy, you also mastermind with other authors who are writing their books, and I want to thank two of them for their help and support. Mike Kitko, who suggested the title *Podiatry Prosperity*, and Alvin Brown. Anyone who thinks they have a book in them but hasn't figured out how to write it should contact Nancy and get started. Her website is www.thebookprofessor.com.

ABOUT THE AUTHOR

Rem Jackson is the CEO and Founder of Top Practices. Since its launch in 2007, Top Practices has helped hundreds of podiatry practices and thousands of doctors and their staff members learn how to market and manage their practices and how to lower the stress of being in business. Rem has earned the American Academy of Podiatric Practice Management's Presidents Award. In 2019, he was inducted into *Podiatry Management's* Podiatric Hall of Fame. He's the proud father of three wonderful daughters. When they aren't visiting all the wine-producing regions of the world, he lives with his best friend and wife, Diane, in Las Vegas, Nevada.

MORE ABOUT TOP PRACTICES

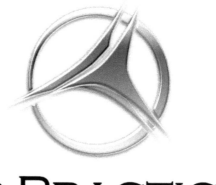

TOP PRACTICES
ACHIEVING PROFESSIONAL GROWTH

The Top Practices Mastermind Group provides executive coaching specifically for podiatrists. It gives them the tools, strategies, and plans to enable them to build their practices into the practices they want. The Top Practices Mastermind Group is also a vibrant community of successful podiatrists and their key staff who share the best ideas, strategies, and tools available to enable them to build and lead highly successful podiatry practices. The members of Top Practices have access to world-class resources 24/7, and specific sessions teaching marketing, management, and a successful business mindset. In addition, members work directly with Rem Jackson as they punch through their action plans and transform their practices. The Mastermind group is for all size practices from the start-up to a multi-doctor, multi-office practice. Members can leave anytime, but most stay for years.

Visit www.TopPractices.com to learn more about the most innovative and respected podiatry business group in existence. We have transformed hundreds of podiatry practices and can transform yours if you are ready. Join us!

JOIN THE TOP PRACTICES VIRTUAL PRACTICE MANAGEMENT INSTITUTE

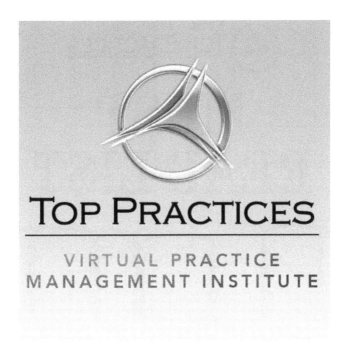

The Top Practices Virtual Practice Management Institute (VPMI), led by Dr. Peter Wishnie and Tina Del Buono, is a breakthrough concept in practice management, coaching, training, and support. Members of the VMPI have 24/7 access to a treasure trove of resources online, covering every issue and challenge medical practices face. Answers, documents, systems, and protocols combined with direct instruction from Dr. Wishnie and Ms. Del Buono provide the most in-depth, comprehensive, and affordable program available anywhere. Members work with our coaches on their action plans as they improve their practices in a step-by-step program. Get your nights and weekends back by managing your practice like a pro.

Visit www.TopPractices.com/Prosperity to learn more about this breakthrough approach to outstanding practice management. If you're ready, your practice can be a dream rather than a nightmare. Please join us!

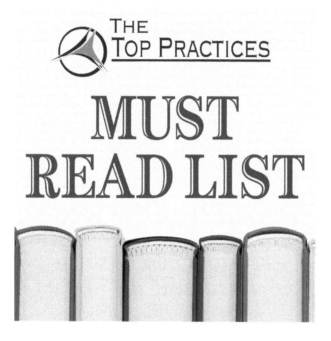

Access the Top Practices Must-Read List at www.TopPractices.com. Rem Jackson has compiled a list of the very best books you can read to build your practice and enhance your mindset and life.